immunology

The National Medical Series for Independent Study

immunology

EDITORS

Richard M. Hyde, Ph.D.

*Department of Microbiology and
    Immunology
University of Oklahoma
    Health Sciences Center
Oklahoma City, Oklahoma*

Robert A. Patnode, Ph.D.

*Department of Microbiology and
    Immunology
University of Oklahoma
    Health Sciences Center
Oklahoma City, Oklahoma*

A WILEY MEDICAL PUBLICATION
JOHN WILEY & SONS
New York • Chichester • Brisbane • Toronto • Singapore

Harwal Publishing Company, Media, Pennsylvania

Library of Congress Cataloging in Publication Data

Immunology.

(The National medical series for independent study)
(A Wiley medical publication)
   Includes index.
   1. Immunology—Outlines, syllabi, etc.   2. Immu-
nology—Examinations, questions, etc.   I. Hyde,
Richard M.   II. Patnode, Robert A.   III. Series.
IV. Series: Wiley medical publication.   [DNLM:
1. Allergy and Immunology—examination questions.
2. Allergy and Immunology—outlines. QW 18 I33]
QR182.55.146   1987   616.07 '9 '076   86-27032
ISBN 0-471-82925-0

©1987 by John Wiley & Sons, Inc.

10 9 8 7 6 5 4 3 2

Contents

Preface

This text was developed as a syllabus to be used in the immunology course taught to second-year medical students at the University of Oklahoma College of Medicine in Oklahoma City. As such, it has been in use since 1975. It has undergone numerous revisions, updatings, and modifications as dictated by student evaluations and developments in the field. In its current form, it is intended to be a synopsis of the most pertinent information available on basic and clinically relevant concepts in immunology. The text first presents a review of native immunity, immunogenicity, the mechanisms and products of immune responses, and practical considerations of immunization and laboratory procedures employed in the diagnosis of disease. The remaining chapters are concerned with defects in native and acquired immunities, with diseases in which the immune system has turned on inappropriately and is autoreactive, and with transplantation and tumor immunology.

This book presents a concise coverage of the fundamentals of immunology in a readily understandable manner. It is hoped that the text will fill the needs of students and former students of immunology who desire a brief, easily readable overview of immunologic fundamentals. To stimulate interest and reinforce the learning process, review questions are presented at the end of each chapter. Relevance of the material to actual clinical situations is illustrated by means of case histories presented in questions in the post-test.

Richard M. Hyde

Preface

Acknowledgments

We would like to express our appreciation to Jim Harris of Harwal Publishing Company, who developed the concept for this series, and to Deborah G. Huey, Project Editor, for her support, guidance, and patience over the months. The assistance of Debra Dreger and Jane Velker in manuscript preparation is also acknowledged. Appreciation is extended to the medical illustrator at Harwal, Wieslawa B. Langenfeld, for development of the illustrations in the text, and to our artist, Dawn Struthers. Special thanks go to Cricket Baughman and Mary Patterson for their tireless efforts in preparing the manuscript.

Many colleagues have contributed to the preparation of this book. Dr. D. Rex Billington served as the catalyst for the preparation of the original manuscript. He contributed innumerable ideas on organization and format, and was invaluable in our efforts to evaluate the teaching effectiveness of the text. Valuable advice on content was obtained from Drs. William A. Cain and Samuel R. Oleinick.

This book is dedicated to the many students, both past and present, who contributed to its preparation through their penetrating questions, thoughtful comments, and constructive criticisms.

Publisher's Note

The objective of the *National Medical Series* is to present an extraordinarily large amount of information in an easily retrievable form. The outline format was selected for this purpose of reducing to the essentials the medical information needed by today's student and practitioner.

While the concept of an outline format was well received by the authors and publisher, the difficulties inherent in working with this style were not initially apparent. That the series has been published and received enthusiastically is a tribute to the authors who worked long and diligently to produce books that are stylistically consistent and comprehensive in content.

The task of producing the *National Medical Series* required more than the efforts of the authors, however, and the missing elements have been supplied by highly competent and dedicated developmental editors and support staff. Editors, compositors, proofreaders, and layout and design staff have all polished the outline to a fine form. It is with deep appreciation that I thank all who have participated, in particular the staff at Harwal—Debra L. Dreger, Jane Edwards, Gloria Hamilton, Deborah G. Huey, Susan Kelly, Wieslawa B. Langenfeld, Keith LaSala, June Sangiorgio Mash, and Jane Velker.

The Publisher

Introduction

Immunology is one of ten basic science review books in the *National Medical Series for Independent Study*. This series has been designed to provide students and house officers, as well as physicians, with a concise but comprehensive instrument for self-evaluation and review within the basic sciences. Although *Immunology* would be most useful for students preparing for the National Board of Medical Examiners examinations (Part I and FLEX) as well as FMGEMS, it should also be useful for students studying for course examinations. These books are not intended to replace the standard basic science texts but, rather, to complement them.

The books in this series present the core content of each basic science, using an outline format and featuring 300 study questions. The questions are distributed throughout the book, at the end of each chapter and in a pretest and post-test. In addition, each question is accompanied by the correct answer, a paragraph-length explanation of the correct answer, and specific reference to the outline points under which the information necessary to answer the question can be found.

We have chosen an outline format to allow maximal ease in retrieving information, assuming that the time available to the reader is limited. Considerable editorial time has been spent to ensure that the information required by all medical school curricula has been included and that the question format parallels that of the National Board examinations. We feel that the combination of the outline and the board-type study questions provides a unique teaching device.

We hope you will find this series interesting, relevant, and challenging. The authors, as well as the John Wiley and Harwal staffs, welcome your comments and suggestions.

Pretest

QUESTIONS

Directions: Each question below contains five suggested answers. Choose the **one best** response to each question.

1. Examples of <u>innate resistance</u> processes include

(A) transplacental passage of IgG
(B) response to vaccination
(C) flushing action of tears
(D) recovery from an infection
(E) administration of antitoxin

2. The secondary immune response

(A) is mainly IgM antibody
(B) requires a low dose of immunogen for induction
(C) has low affinity antibodies
(D) has a short duration of antibody synthesis
(E) has a slow rate of antibody synthesis

3. An <u>antigen</u> should possess two properties. These are

(A) chemical simplicity and immunogenicity
(B) allergenicity and immunogenicity
(C) toxicity and allergenicity
(D) toxicity and specific reactivity
(E) immunogenicity and specific reactivity

4. Persons with <u>hereditary angioedema</u> have a deficiency in

(A) C3b inactivator
(B) C1 esterase inhibitor
(C) C5 convertase
(D) properdin
(E) C3 activator

5. In the generation of atopic hypersensitivity, fixation of IgE to mast cells and basophils occurs via the

(A) Fc fragment
(B) C1 domain
(C) Fab fragment
(D) C2 domain
(E) V region

6. In the classical pathway of complement activation, C1 esterase mediates cleavage of

(A) C1
(B) C2
(C) C3
(D) C4
(E) C5

7. Immunodeficiency resulting in increased susceptibility to <u>viral and fungal infections</u> is due primarily to a deficiency in

(A) macrophages
(B) B cells
(C) T cells
(D) neutrophils
(E) complement

8. The test used to detect the presence of circulating <u>nonagglutinating antibody</u> is the

(A) liquid-phase radioimmunoassay (RIA)
(B) indirect Coombs test
(C) Rose-Waaler test
(D) Schick test
(E) complement fixation test

1

9. A 4-year-old child suffering from repeated infections with staphylococci and streptococci was found to have normal phagocytic function and delayed hypersensitivity responses. Lymph node biopsy would probably reveal

(A) depletion of thymus-dependent regions
(B) intact germinal centers
(C) hyperplastic degeneration
(D) lack of plasma cells
(E) normal serum immunoglobulin levels

10. All of the following are neutrophil defects that could result in immunodeficiency EXCEPT

(A) impaired chemotaxis
(B) insufficient hexose monophosphate shunt (glucose) metabolism
(C) suppression of intracellular killing
(D) abnormal complement levels
(E) defective opsonization

11. A substance that can evoke either a humoral or a cell-mediated immune response is termed

(A) an immunogen
(B) a hapten
(C) an epitope
(D) an antigen
(E) an adjuvant

12. In a child with severe combined immunodeficiency disease (SCID), the most important complication of treatment by bone marrow transplantation is

(A) malignant transformation of the transplanted cells
(B) failure to develop isohemagglutinins
(C) graft-versus-host reaction
(D) rejection of the transplanted tissue
(E) lack of mature B cells in the bone marrow graft

13. B-cell membranes contain receptors for all of the following EXCEPT

(A) Fc portion of immunoglobulin
(B) lipopolysaccharide
(C) endotoxin
(D) concanavalin A
(E) pokeweed mitogen

14. Renal failure is a common cause of death in patients with

(A) Sjögren's syndrome
(B) rheumatoid arthritis
(C) rheumatic fever
(D) pemphigus vulgaris
(E) systemic lupus erythematosus

15. Immune tolerance can be described as being

(A) specific to each epitope on a particular antigen
(B) most easily induced in adult animals
(C) synonymous with autotolerance
(D) enhanced by the use of adjuvants
(E) blocked by the drug cyclophosphamide

16. Which of the following serologic tests would be the most valuable in confirmation of a suspected case of infectious mononucleosis?

(A) Quantitative radial immunodiffusion
(B) Coombs test
(C) Sheep red blood cell (SRBC) agglutinins
(D) Weil-Felix OX-19 test
(E) Weil-Felix OX-2 test

17. Toxoids are best described as being

(A) immunogenic and toxic
(B) nonimmunogenic and toxic
(C) immunogenic and nontoxic
(D) nonimmunogenic and nontoxic
(E) neither antigenic nor immunogenic

18. Sera used for HLA typing by cytotoxicity assay are obtained from all of the following sources EXCEPT

(A) multiparous women
(B) rabbits immunized with human lymphocytes
(C) patients who have received many blood transfusions
(D) patients who have received and rejected tranplanted grafts
(E) volunteers who have been HLA sensitized

19. Rheumatoid factor is an antibody directed against determinants on the

(A) gamma chain
(B) mu chain
(C) J chain
(D) lambda chain
(E) kappa chain

20. A 7-month-old child was hospitalized for a yeast infection that would not respond to therapy. He had a history of acute pyogenic infections. Examination of the patient revealed lymphopenia, absence of thymus shadow on x-ray, hypogammaglobulinemia, and lack of B cells. This history is most compatible with

(A) acquired immune deficiency syndrome (AIDS)
(B) multiple myeloma
(C) chronic granulomatous disease (CGD)
(D) Bruton's X-linked hypogammaglobulinemia
(E) severe combined immunodeficiency disease (SCID)

21. The predominant antibody in saliva is

(A) IgA
(B) IgG
(C) IgM
(D) IgD
(E) IgE

Directions: Each question below contains four suggested answers of which **one or more** is correct. Choose the answer

    A   if **1, 2, and 3** are correct
    B   if **1 and 3** are correct
    C   if **2 and 4** are correct
    D   if **4** is correct
    E   if **1, 2, 3, and 4** are correct

22. True statements describing cell-mediated immunity include

(1) antilymphocyte serum suppresses its expression
(2) humoral antibody is bound to the cells
(3) following antigen injection, skin reactions of sensitive persons are visible within 48 hours
(4) cortisone enhances its expression

23. The diversity generating gene segment D is present in

(1) delta domain DNA
(2) light chain genes
(3) lambda domain DNA
(4) heavy chain genes

24. Antigenic markers of immunoglobulin molecules referred to as Km are

(1) associated with kappa light chains
(2) genetically determined
(3) allotypic determinants
(4) associated with gamma heavy chains

25. T cells are involved in

(1) production of interleukin-2
(2) acquired resistance to tuberculosis
(3) contact dermatitis
(4) response to interleukin-1

26. Hypervariable regions of IgG molecules exist on

(1) Fc fragment
(2) heavy chain
(3) C_L domain
(4) light chain

27. Although the mammalian counterpart of the avian bursa of Fabricius is unknown, candidates include

(1) spleen
(2) gut-associated lymphoid tissue (GALT)
(3) thymus
(4) bone marrow

28. Adjuvants are nonspecific substances that are sometimes used to

(1) enhance antibody synthesis
(2) induce immune tolerance
(3) enhance immune response
(4) remove antibodies from the circulation

29. Assays of immune competence involve the evaluation of

(1) T cells
(2) B cells
(3) phagocytic cells
(4) innate immunity

SUMMARY OF DIRECTIONS

A	B	C	D	E
1, 2, 3 only	1, 3 only	2, 4 only	4 only	All are correct

30. Assays used for the detection of immune complexes in serum include

(1) enzyme-linked immunosorbent assay (ELISA)
(2) Raji cell binding assay
(3) liquid-phase radioimmunoassay (RIA)
(4) C1q solid-phase binding assay

31. Treatment of the IgG monomer with papain splits it into

(1) one F(ab')$_2$ fragment
(2) two Fab fragments
(3) two Fd fragments
(4) one Fc fragment

32. Tests for measuring phagocytic function include

(1) microbicidal activity
(2) nitroblue tetrazolium reduction
(3) chemiluminescence
(4) chemotaxis

33. True statements concerning antigens involved in transplantation include

(1) because red blood cell (ABO) antigens appear on tissue cells, they function as transplantation antigens
(2) because HLA antigens appear on granulocytes, lymphocytes, and platelets, incompatibility for these antigens in certain recipients of whole blood can cause febrile transfusion reactions
(3) blood transfusion, pregnancy, and previous skin or organ transplants can sensitize individuals to histocompatibility antigens
(4) no new immune response occurs in tissue transplanted between antigenically identical individuals

34. Characteristic differences between innate and adaptive immunity include

(1) induction
(2) specificity
(3) immunologic memory
(4) phagocytosis

35. The human major histocompatibility complex (MHC) has genes that code for

(1) antigens on the surface of B cells and macrophages
(2) certain complement components
(3) antigens that may elicit antibody formation in unrelated persons
(4) variable domains of immunoglobulin molecules

36. Tumor-specific transplantation antigens (TSTAs) are a subpopulation of tumor-specific antigens (TSAs) that occur on the membrane of the tumor cell. TSTAs may possibly

(1) induce an antibody response
(2) have a viral etiology
(3) elicit cytotoxic T (Tc) cell responses
(4) induce suppressor T (Ts) cells

37. Immunoglobulin molecules contain

(1) heavy and light chains
(2) domains
(3) hinge regions
(4) phagosomes

38. DPT vaccine is used to induce protection against

(1) typhoid fever
(2) whooping cough
(3) dengue
(4) tetanus

39. Immune tolerance can be induced by

(1) adult thymectomy
(2) neonatal thymectomy
(3) excess antibody
(4) excess antigen

Directions: For each numbered item below, select the one lettered choice with which it is most closely associated. Each lettered choice may be used once, more than once, or not at all. Choose the answer

> **A** if the item is associated with **(A) only**
> **B** if the item is associated with **(B) only**
> **C** if the item is associated with **both (A) and (B)**
> **D** if the item is associated with **neither (A) nor (B)**

40. Examples of cancer-associated antigens that probably arise from tissue dedifferentiation include

(A) carcinoembryonic antigen (CEA)
(B) alpha-fetoprotein
(C) both
(D) neither

41. Antiviral products from macrophage lysosomes include

(A) interferon
(B) lysozyme
(C) both
(D) neither

42. Neutrophil membranes contain receptors for

(A) Fc fragment of IgG
(B) C3b
(C) both
(D) neither

ultraviolet Radiation → Thymine dimer.

43. Ionizing radiation is most efficient in suppressing

(A) ongoing immune responses
(B) the induction of an immune response
(C) both are equally sensitive to radiation
(D) neither are suppressed by radiation

44. Vaccines induce immunity that is

(A) active artificially acquired immunity
(B) passive artificially acquired immunity
(C) both
(D) neither

45. Oxygen-independent antimicrobial systems of the macrophage include

(A) transferrin
(B) hypochlorite
(C) both
(D) neither

46. Class II HLA antigens are immune response-associated (Ia) antigens characterized by

(A) their presence on most nucleated cells in humans
(B) their structural similarity to the antigen-binding (Fab) fragment of an immunoglobulin molecule
(C) both
(D) neither

Directions: The groups of questions below consist of lettered choices followed by several numbered items. For each numbered item select the **one** lettered choice with which it is **most** closely associated. Each lettered choice may be used once, more than once, or not at all.

Questions 47–50

For each characteristic, select the disorder most closely associated with it.

(A) Guillain-Barré syndrome
(B) Systemic lupus erythematosus
(C) Sjögren's syndrome
(D) Goodpasture's syndrome
(E) Acute disseminated encephalomyelitis

47. Dry eyes and dry mouth

48. Peripheral neuritis

49. Antibody specific for antigen shared by kidney and lung

50. Butterfly rash

Questions 51–55

Match the pathologic feature with the disorder with which it is most closely associated.

(A) Multiple myeloma
(B) Allergic rhinitis
(C) Arthus reaction
(D) Serum sickness
(E) Idiopathic thrombocytopenic purpura (ITP)

51. Strong hereditary association

52. Platelet-specific IgG antibodies on platelet surfaces

53. Local immune complex deposition

54. Systemic immune complex deposition

55. Bence Jones protein in the urine

Questions 56–60

For each characteristic of a complement component, select the component it best describes.

(A) C3b,B
(B) C3a
(C) C3
(D) Bb
(E) C5b6789

56. Destroyed by anaphylotoxin inactivator

57. Membrane attack complex

58. Binds to $\overline{C4b2a}$ complex

59. Cleaved by factor $\overline{D}$

60. Activates macrophages and causes them to adhere to and spread on surfaces.

ANSWERS AND EXPLANATIONS

1. The answer is C. (*Chapter 1 I A, B 1; Table 1-1*) Innate immunities are those which are present in the absence of any antigenic exposure. The flushing action of tears is an example of innate resistance. This process is active and independent of antigen exposure, regardless of prior microbial encounters. Transplacental passage of IgG, on the other hand, is a naturally acquired immunity that is of an active immunologic basis (e.g., maternal synthesis of antibodies in response to a specific antigenic challenge; these antibodies cross the placenta and afford the fetus passive protection). This, as well as recovery from disease, is a natural process, but it is not an innate immunity. Vaccination is an example of active artifically acquired immunity and administration of antitoxin is an example of passive artificially acquired immunity.

2. The answer is B. (*Chapter 5 IV A 2, 3*) The secondary immune response, also referred to as the booster or anamnestic response, is triggered by relatively low doses of immunogen. The secondary immune response is mainly IgG antibody, and the antibodies produced are of high affinity for the antigen. Another feature of the secondary immune response is a rapid rate of production of antibody, usually accompanied by an antibody level which exceeds the previous, or primary, immune response.

3. The answer is E. (*Chapter 2 I A*) Antigens must be both immunogenic and specifically reactive. They need not induce allergies (allergenicity) and should not be toxic, although toxicity is not a feature which would preclude antigenicity.

4. The answer is B. (*Chapter 11 VII A*) Hereditary angioedema is an inherited defect characterized by transient but recurrent local (e.g., skin, gastrointestinal tract, respiratory tract) edema. The patients have a deficiency of C$\bar{1}$ esterase inhibitor which leads to uncontrolled C1 esterase activity and resultant production of a kinin which increases capillary permeability.

5. The answer is A. (*Chapter 3 II C, D, E 1 a b; III E 2 d; Chapter 9 II B*) In the generation of atopic hypersensitivity, antigen (allergen)-specific IgE is produced which is described as homocytotropic due to its affinity for cells ("cytotropic") of the host species that produced it ("homo"), particularly for tissue mast cells and blood basophils. Cell adherence occurs via the Fc fragment (C3 and C4 domains).

6. The answer is D. (*Chapter 4 II A 2 a, b*) In the classical pathway of complement activation the first component to bind is C$\bar{1}$ which acquires esterase activity and is referred to as C1 esterase. The latter then mediates cleavage of C4 into C4a and C4b. C4b can bind to cell membranes; C4a is released into the fluid phase and acts as an anaphylatoxin.

7. The answer is C. (*Chapter 11 IV A*) Profoundly impaired T-cell function, such as that seen in DiGeorge syndrome, manifests itself by recurrent infection with viral, fungal, as well as protozoan and certain intracellular bacterial pathogens. Protection against such agents depends largely on intact cell (T cell)-mediated immunity.

8. The answer is B. (*Chapter 8 III E 2*) The indirect Coombs test is used to detect circulating nonagglutinating antibody; for example, it is valuable in detecting IgG-associated antibody in the serum of a woman who is believed to be sensitized to the Rh antigen and is at risk for carrying an erythroblastotic fetus. The Schick test is used to test for immunity to diphtheria. The complement fixation test, Rose-Waaler test, and liquid-phase radioimmunoassay (RIA) are different techniques used to measure antigen–antibody reactions.

9. The answer is D. (*Chapter 11 III A*) The child described in the question probably has Bruton's X-linked hypogammaglobulinemia which manifests as recurrent infections with such organisms as staphylococci and streptococci and is associated with a B-cell deficiency. Features of the disease include lack of germinal centers and plasma cells in lymph nodes, low serum levels of immunoglobulins, intact T-cell (thymus) and phagocytic function, and absent or hypoplastic tonsils and Peyer's patches.

10. The answer is D. [*Chapter 11 II B 1 a (2), b*] In qualitative immunodeficiency disorders, the phagocytic cells are involved; B-cell, T-cell, and complement levels and functions are generally normal. Neutrophil immunodeficiency could be due to a defect in any of the processes involved in neutrophil protective action. A defect in chemotaxis that would block phagocytic cell ability to migrate to the site of inflammation could cause immune deficiency. Also, a defect in opsonization, or a defect in phagocytosis or degranulation of the lysosome could result in defective neutrophil function. If the hexose monophosphate shunt activity is insufficient, there would not be the energy in the cell required for chemotaxis or new membrane synthesis, which are essential parts of phagocytosis. Intracellular killing defects could be due to the absence of enzymes which are needed for killing, or the absence of oxygen-dependent or oxygen-independent microbicidal activities.

11. The answer is A. (*Chapter 2 I A 1, 2*) Immunogenic materials are those which are able to induce an immune response when administered to an animal to which they are foreign. The response may be humoral (i.e., circulating antibodies) or it may be a cell-mediated immune response (i.e., the production of specifically sensitized lymphocytes).

12. The answer is C. (*Chapter 11 V A 2; Chapter 12 II B 2 b*) The major problem in bone marrow transplantation is the incorporation in the transplant of viable lymphoid cells. These cells could mount a graft-versus-host reaction in the recipient. This is particularly true if the recipient's immune system is compromised, as in the case of a combined immunodeficiency, or in the case of a transplant individual under immunosuppression.

13. The answer is D. (*Chapter 5 V B 3 b*) B-cell membranes contain receptors for pokeweed mitogen, as well as lipopolysaccharides such as the endotoxin of gram-negative bacteria. These molecules will induce mitosis in the B cell. This mitosis can be quantitated by measuring the incorporation of tritiated thymidine into the DNA of the cells. Thus the amount of B-cell activity can be quantitated. B cells also contain an Fc receptor in their membrane. Receptors for phytohemagglutinin and concanavalin A are contained in the T-cell membranes.

14. The answer is E. [*Chapter 10 V H 1 b (2)*] Systemic lupus erythematosus is a chronic, systemic inflammatory, multiorgan disease triggered by the deposition of immune complexes on basement membrane of blood vessels. Renal failure is a common cause of death since immune complex deposition commonly occurs in blood vessels of renal glomeruli, leading to development of glomerulonephritis.

15. The answer is A. [*Chapter 6 II B 2; III B 7, 8 a, 9 a; IV A*] Each epitope reacts with specific T-cell and B-cell clones, and each clone must be blocked or deleted before total immune tolerance can be achieved. Anything less would result in partial tolerance or split tolerance. Tolerance is most easily induced in neonates or after immunosuppression by such drugs as cyclophosphamide. Adjuvants enhance immune responses and hence would actually interfere with tolerance induction.

16. The answer is C. (*Chapter 2 II A 4 b; Chapter 8 II C 3, III E*) Infectious mononucleosis can be diagnosed by the presence in the patient's serum of antibodies which agglutinate sheep erythrocytes. These antibodies are directed to an antigen on the erythrocyte which is shared with the infectious mononucleosis virus (the Epstein-Barr virus). This is a heterophilic antigen relationship, and the test used to detect it is the Paul-Bunnell hemagglutination procedure. Infectious mononucleosis caused by another herpes virus, cytomegalovirus, is not accompanied by the production of sheep erythrocyte agglutinins.

Rickettsial infections induce in the affected individual the agglutination of certain strains of *Proteus vulgaris*, a heterophilic immune response termed the Weil-Felix reaction. Quantitative radial immunodiffusion is useful in determination of hypergammaglobulinemic or hypogammaglobulinemic states. The Coombs test is used to detect antibodies in a person's serum reactive with erythrocytes. In a case of erythroblastosis fetalis, or in a transfusion reaction, the Coombs test might be used to identify the nature of the antibody involved in the disease process.

17. The answer is C. (*Chapter 7 II A 2 b*) Toxins of several bacteria can be converted into nontoxic but still immunogenic preparations called toxoids. Heat or formalin can be used for their preparation. Toxoids make excellent vaccines for the purpose of inducing active immunity.

18. The answer is B. (*Chapter 12 II C 1*) The sera employed in the cytotoxicity test used to identify HLA antigens is obtained from multiparous women, patients who have received and rejected allografts, patients who have received multiple transfusions, and volunteers who have been HLA sensitized by blood transfusions, white cell inoculations, or tissue grafts. All of these people would be sensitized to HLA antigens, the antigens being unique to the fetus, the graft, or the transfused lymphocytes. Such sensitization would result in the production of antibodies specific for the particular HLA antigen to which the person has been exposed. Rabbits immunized with human lymphocytes would produce an array of antibodies to lymphocytes, which would not have the epitope specificity needed for the cytotoxicity assay.

19. The answer is A. (*Chapter 10 V H 2 a 1, 2*) Rheumatoid factor is an antibody that has specificity for the gamma immunoglobulin heavy chain. It is usually of the IgM class; however, rheumatoid factors have also been described which are IgG or IgA. These molecules occur in a high percentage (70%–90%) of patients with rheumatoid arthritis. Other autoimmune diseases also will induce rheumatoid factor in the patient's sera (e.g., systemic lupus erythematosus and Sjögren's syndrome). Rheumatoid factor is found in patients with leprosy, tuberculosis, and other nonautoimmune diseases.

20. The answer is E. (*Chapter 11 V A*) Severe combined immunodeficiency disease (SCID) involves a combined defect in both humoral (B-cell–mediated) and cell (T-cell)–mediated immunity as evidenced by lymphopenia, absence of thymus shadow on x-ray, hypogammaglobulinemia, and lack of B cells or antibody response. Patients usually die within the first year or two of life from viral, bacterial, fungal, or protozoan infection. \

21. The answer is A. (*Chapter 1 III C 2*) While some immunoglobulin G (IgG) and IgM can be found in gingival pocket fluid, IgA predominates in saliva. IgG is the major antibody in the serum. IgM is the first antibody synthesized in utero and during postnatal antibody responses. IgE is the immunoglobulin associated with anaphylaxis and atopic diseases such as asthma and hay fever. IgD globulin has been connected to antibody activity (e.g., hypersensitivity to penicillin in humans).

22. The answer is B (1,3). [*Chapter 6 II B 2 a, b (4), c (1) (b); Chapter 8 IV C 2 a (1) (3)*] Cell-mediated, or T-cell, immunity can be suppressed by antilymphocyte sera. Cell-mediated immunity is involved in tumor rejection. It is also involved in resistance to certain viral, fungal, and mycobacterial pathogens. Individuals who have a positive skin test to purified protein derivative (PPD) of the tubercle bacillus will react with an area of induration of 10 mm or greater 48 hours after exposure to that antigen. T cells do not have antibody bound to their membranes; they are also sensitive to cortisone suppression.

23. The answer is D (4). (*Chapter 3 IV B 4 a–c*) Heavy chain gene organization, although similar to that of light chain genes, is more complex in that three, not two, segments of DNA join together to generate the variable portion of the heavy chain. The additional segment is designated the diversity (D_H) gene region.

24. The answer is A (1, 2, 3). (*Chapter 3 IV A 1*) Allotypes are genetic markers on heavy and light immunoglobulin chains that are inherited in a mendelian fashion and are usually localized in the constant region. Allotypic markers found in kappa light chains are designated Km.

25. The answer is E (all). [*Chapter 5; Chapter 9 V C 1 c (1)*] T cells are involved in contact dermatitis and are effector cells in tuberculosis immunity. In addition, T cells respond to interleukin-1 produced by antigen-presenting macrophages and will produce interleukin-2 in response to that hormonal signal.

26. The answer is C (2, 4). (*Chapter 3 II C 1 a, b*) The variable (V) regions of heavy (H) and light (L) chains of immunoglobulin molecules have areas of high variability called hypervariable regions ("hot spots"), which are most intimately involved in formation of the antigen-binding site. There are three to four hypervariable regions in both V_H and V_L regions (hv1–hv3).

27. The answer is C (2, 4). (*Chapter 5 II B 2 b*) The avian bursa of Fabricius is an organ responsible for the maturation of the B-cell component of the immune system. The mammalian counterpart of this avian organ is unknown; however, gut-associated lymphoid tissues have been implicated. The bone marrow has been suggested as a possible location wherein the B cells may obtain their immunologic education. The thymus is the organ (in birds as well as in mammals) which is responsible for maturation and differentiation of the T cells of the immune system. Splenectomy will decrease the antibody content of serum transiently, but would not cause permanent immunosuppression.

28. The answer is B (1, 3). (*Chapter 6 IV A 1 a, b*) Adjuvants are nonspecific, mildly irritating substances that are used to enhance antibody synthesis. They act as a depot for the slow release of antigen through the reticuloendothelial system (RES) of the animal being immunized. Some adjuvants have an irritant action that also enhances the immune response.

29. The answer is E (all). (*Chapter 1 I A; Chapter 8 IV*) T cells, B cells, and phagocytic cells are all evaluated in order to assess immune competence. Various assays, tests, and techniques are used in analyzing the cells. Phagocytic cells are analyzed by using assays for testing the metabolism and generation of toxic molecules, the ingestion and killing of microorganisms, and chemotaxis. Analysis of B cells and T cells involves the enumeration of pre-B cells, T-cell subsets, as well as B cells and T cells that are present in an individual; and determining whether these cells are functional. Innate immunity refers to the naturally occurring, nonspecific defense mechanisms that protect an individual from infectious diseases, including phagocytosis.

30. The answer is C (2, 4). (*Chapter 8 III G 1, H 1 a, b; IV B 2 e*) Assays available for detecting immune complexes in serum and other biologic fluids can be divided into solid-phase binding assays, liquid-phase binding assays, and cellular binding assays. C1q solid-phase and liquid-phase binding assays are techniques used to evaluate the complement component C1q, which has an affinity for immune complexes, thus allowing recognition of immune complexes. Raji cells, a human lymphoblastoid cell line, are used in a binding assay based on the ability of immune complexes to bind to the Raji cells through

C3 receptors. The immune complexes bound to the surface of the Raji cells can be assayed by the addition of radiolabeled anti-IgG antibody. Enzyme-linked immunosorbent assay (ELISA) and liquid-phase radioimmunoassay (RIA) are not used in the evaluation of immune complexes. RIA is an extremely sensitive method used to quantitate any immunogenic or haptenic substance that can be labeled with a radioactive isotope (e.g., iodine 125). ELISA has about the same sensitivity as RIA and is used to assay both antigens and antibodies via attachment to a solid-phase support (e.g., plastic surfaces) or linkage to an enzyme (e.g., horseradish peroxidase).

31. The answer is C (2, 4). (*Chapter 3 II E 1 a, b*) Treatment of the monomeric basic immunoglobulin unit with the enzyme papain splits it into two monovalent Fab (antigen-binding) fragments, each containing an entire light chain and the V_H and C_H1 domains of the heavy chain (Fd fragment), and one Fc (crystallizable) fragment containing the carboxy terminal half of the heavy chains.

32. The answer is E (all). (*Chapter 1 II C 4 a, c, d, e*) Tests for measuring phagocytic function include microbicidal activity, nitroblue tetrazolium reduction, chemiluminescence, and chemotaxis. Intracellular killing by phagocytic cells can be measured by direct plate counting of mixtures of microorganisms and cells, or by the use of supravital stains such as acridine orange to assess the viability of engulfed microbes. Nitroblue tetrazolium is a yellow, water-soluble dye that converts to a purple, water-insoluble intracellular compound called formazan when phagocytizing neutrophils produce hydrogen peroxide and superoxide anion during the phagocytic process. Chemiluminescence is used to measure the light produced by singlet oxygen, a microbicidal compound generated by oxygen-dependent mechanisms within the lysosomal granules that are responsible for destroying foreign particles.

33. The answer is E (all). [*Chapter 12 I A; II C 1 b (2), D 1*] All of the statements in the question are correct. The ABO antigens are very potent transplantation antigens, and incompatibility between donor and recipient results in hyperacute rejection. The presence of HLA antigens on white blood cells and platelets can cause HLA sensitization and febrile reactions upon secondary exposure.

34. The answer is A (1, 2, 3). (*Chapter 1 I A, B; Chapter 5 IV A 3*) The three characteristic differences between innate and adaptive (or acquired) immunity are the presence of an induction phase, the immunologic specificity of adaptive, acquired immune mechanisms, and the immunologic memory that the system demonstrates. Immunologic memory is the anamnestic response, wherein a more rapid production of antibody to a higher level is achieved upon secondary antigenic exposure.

35. The answer is A (1, 2, 3). (*Chapter 12 II B 2, 3, 4*) The human major histocompatibility complex (MHC) is composed of a cluster of genes located on chromosome 6, which code for three (and possibly four) distinct classes of molecules. Class I and class II MHC molecules are important for controlling immunologic defense. The MHC-encoded class I antigens (HLA-A, HLA-B, HLA-C) can be expressed on all human nucleated cells. MHC-encoded class II antigens (HLA-D/DR antigens), which are also called immune response–associated (Ia) antigens, can be expressed on the surface of immunocompetent cells, principally B cells and macrophages. Class II antigens are important in the cellular recognition that permits the cellular interaction needed to induce an immune response. Class III molecules are certain complement components (C4, C2, factor B of the alternative pathway) encoded by genes in the MHC. Class IV molecules have been identified as components of the H-2 system in mice and are believed to exist as such in humans but, as yet, have not been fully characterized.

36. The answer is E (all). (*Chapter 13 II A 2 b; B 2; C 1, 2*) Viruses may specify tumor-specific transplantation antigens (TSTAs) which will appear on the membrane of the tumor (transformed) cell. TSTAs may induce an antibody response, they may induce the development in the host of cytotoxic T (Tc) cells, or they may induce suppressor T (Ts) cells. Tumor development may be a bypass of immune surveillance, a mechanism by which the body continuously purges itself of potentially cancerous cells. Factors that decrease immune capabilities predispose an individual to malignancy.

37. The answer is A (1, 2, 3). (*Chapter 1 II C 2 c; Chapter 3 II A, D, F*) All classes (isotypes) of immunoglobulins contain heavy chains, light chains, domains, and hinge regions. A phagosome is an intracellular phagocytic vesicle.

38. The answer is C (2, 4). (*Chapter 7 II C; III A 3 a*) DPT vaccine consists of toxoids of diphtheria (precipitated with potassium alum or adsorbed onto aluminum hydroxide or phosphate) and tetanus (adsorbed) combined with killed *Bordetella pertussis*; it is used to protect against diphtheria, tetanus, and pertussis (whooping cough). It is recommended for active immunization of children in a five-dose schedule at age 2 months, 4 months, 6 months, 15–19 months, and 4–6 years (school entry). Dengue is a mosquito-borne viral infection for which vaccine has been prepared but is not included in the DPT vaccine. There is a polyvalent, killed bacterial vaccine which is used throughout the world to prevent typhoid fever.

39. The answer is D (4). (*Chapter 6 III B 1, 3*) There is an antigen threshold that must be reached before an immune response can be induced. There is also an upper limit and if this is exceeded, immune tolerance can result. The form of the antigen is also important. Aggregated antigens are usually quite immunogenic, whereas monomeric forms of the same protein are tolerogenic.

40. The answer is C. [*Chapter 13 II B 1 a (1) (2) (3), b (1) (2)*] Carcinoembryonic antigen (CEA) and alpha-fetoprotein are both antigens which are common in dedifferentiated tissues. They are found in fetal life and in certain malignancies. CEA is associated with cancer of the colon. Alpha-fetoprotein is associated with primary hepatic carcinoma. Other conditions will cause these antigens to appear in the serum (e.g., pregnancy, heavy cigarette smoking, and various infectious diseases). Consequently, they cannot be used diagnostically for the detection of cancer.

41. The answer is A. [*Chapter 1 II C 2 d (2) (a) (iii), D 2 d*] Interferon is an antiviral protein produced by cells of the body in response to viral infection or in response to polynucleotides that have been ingested or pinocytosed. These polynucleotides induce in the cell the production of proteins which interfere with the replication of viruses. Interferon induces cells to make products which inhibit viral replication. These products include a specific RNAse and inhibitors of RNA and protein synthesis. Lysozyme, the product found in the macrophage lysosome, is effective as an antibacterial agent as it causes the breakdown of peptidoglycan.

42. The answer is C. [*Chapter 3 III A 2 c, e; Chapter 4 II A 1 a, 2 d (1), B 2 a*] Neutrophil membranes contain receptors for the Fc fragment of IgG and the Fc fragment of IgM. In addition, they have receptors for C3b. These molecules are referred to as opsonins (e.g., they enhance phagocytosis of foreign materials). An antibody which has reacted on the surface, such as a bacterium, would have the Fc fragment sticking away from the organism. Complement might be activated and the C3b molecule would also be attached to that bacterial cell surface. The neutrophil membrane receptors interacting with that Fc fragment of the antibody molecule or the C3b molecule, would then be in firm union with the particle to be engulfed.

43. The answer is B. (*Chapter 6 II B 2 a*) Ongoing immune responses are, as a rule, refractory to immunosuppression. The induction of immune responses, on the other hand, are usually susceptible to immunosuppression. Ionizing radiation is a cytotoxic treatment that kills rapidly dividing cells. In the induction of an immune response, it is necessary for B cells and T cells to divide. Agents such as ionizing radiation, purine and pyrimidine analogs, and folic acid antagonists that block DNA synthesis will block the induction of a response. Ongoing immune responses (e.g., the production of antibody) do not depend on cell division; therefore, agents such as ionizing radiation are not suppressive.

44. The answer is A. (*Chapter 1 I B; Chapter 7 I B*) Vaccines induce active artificially acquired immunity. Naturally acquired active immunity would be that immunity acquired as a result of recovering from disease. Passive artificially acquired immunity would result from administration of preformed antibody, whereas naturally acquired passive immunity would be that gained by an infant via placental transfer of antibody from the mother.

45. The answer is A. (*Chapter 1 II C 3 b, D 2 e*) Transferrin is an antimicrobial system of the macrophage which is active independent of oxygen presence in the environment. Transferrin is a protein which chelates iron, thus competing with the microbe for this essential cation. Hypochlorite killing is an oxygen-dependent process requiring myeloperoxidase enzyme, hydrogen peroxide, and a halide, in this case a chloride ion.

46. The answer is B. (*Chapter 3 II D 1, 2, E 1 a; Chapter 12 II B 3 a*) Class I HLA antigens are found on the surfaces of most nucleated cells and platelets in humans; class II HLA antigens are found predominantly on the cells involved in the immune response, including macrophages, monocytes, resting T cells, activated T cells, and, particularly, B cells. In mice the class II H-2 antigens are also found on red blood cells. Class II antigens are similar in structure to the antigen-binding fragment (Fab) of antibody; both have two chains of two extracellular domains each.

47–50. The answers are: 47-C, 48-A, 49-D, 50-B. [*Chapter 10 V J 1 a, F 1 b, M 1 a 2 b, H 1 b (1)*] Sjögren's syndrome is a chronic inflammatory disease that affects, primarily, secretory glands such as the lacrimal and salivary glands producing dry eyes (keratoconjunctivitis) and dry mouth (xerostomia).

Guillain-Barré syndrome (acute idiopathic polyneuritis) manifests itself as progressive weakness, first of the lower extremities, and then of the upper extremities and respiratory muscles. Peripheral nerve tissue shows perivascular mononuclear cell infiltrate and demyelination.

Goodpasture's syndrome is a relatively rare disorder with symptoms referrable to both the lungs (e.g., pulmonary hemorrhage) and kidneys (e.g., glomerulonephritis). The IgG immunoglobulin deposited on alveolar and glomerular basement membranes appears to be antibody-specific for an antigen shared by the kidneys and lungs.

Systemic lupus erythematosus is a chronic, systemic, inflammatory multiorgan disease that affects primarily females. Death usually results from renal failure or infection. A characteristic feature is the erythematous "butterfly" rash that occurs on the face of some patients.

51–55. The answers are: 51-B, 52-E, 53-C, 54-D, 55-A. (*Chapter 9 II B 4; III C 2 c; IV C 1, 2; VI A; Chapter 10 V B 8*) The same immunologic mechanisms that defend the host at times may cause severe damage to tissues. These damaging immunologic reactions, sometimes referred to as hypersensitivity reactions, have been classified into four types: immediate hypersensitivity (type I) reactions; cytotoxic (type II) reactions; immune complex–mediated (type III) reactions; and delayed hypersensitivity (cell-mediated; type IV) reactions. Tissue damage also may be caused by immunoglobulin excess that is due to any of the several plasma cell dyscrasias.

Immediate hypersensitivity reactions are initiated by antigens reacting with cell-bound IgE antibody. The reaction may manifest in many ways, ranging from life-threatening systemic anaphylaxis to the lesser disturbances of atopic allergies, such as allergic rhinitis (hay fever), urticaria (hives), and food allergies. Atopic allergies occur only in genetically predisposed hosts upon sensitization to specific allergens. They also show a strong hereditary association; if both parents are atopic, it is probable that their children also will be atopic.

Cytotoxic reactions are initiated by IgG or IgM antibody reacting with antigenic determinants on cell membranes or tissues. The ultimate effect of these reactions is lysis or inactivation of target cells. Idiopathic thrombocytopenic purpura (ITP) is a platelet disorder that occurs by such a mechanism, that is, antibody-mediated destruction of platelets. ITP patients reveal platelet-specific IgG antibodies on platelet surfaces, profoundly suppressed peripheral blood platelet counts, and various bleeding problems.

Immune complex-mediated reactions are initiated by antigen–antibody complexes that form locally or in the circulation and deposit in vascular or glomerular basement membrane where they cause inflammation. The Arthus reaction and serum sickness are classic examples of immune complex disease associated with local and systemic deposition of immune complexes, respectively. The Arthus reaction, induced in rabbits via repeated subcutaneous injections of antigen, is characterized by local foci of erythema, edema, and necrosis at injection sites, which are related to a vasculitis caused by immune complex deposition on vascular basement membrane. Serum sickness refers to the syndrome that follows injection of foreign serum into humans. It is characterized by fever, rash, splenomegaly, arthritis, and glomerulonephritis, and the primary damage—as in the Arthus reaction—appears to be a vasculitis associated with destruction of vascular basement membrane.

Multiple myeloma, the most common of the plasma cell dyscrasias, is a plasma cell tumor in bone marrow that overproduces a single class of immunoglobulins. The most characteristic feature of multiple myeloma is the demonstration of an abnormal protein (M protein) in blood, urine, or both. The M protein usually consists of any one or a combination of heavy (H) chains, IgG, IgA, and light (L) chains. M proteins consisting of only L chains are demonstrated in 25% of cases and only appear in the urine. Bence-Jones protein, a dimer of immunoglobulin L chains, is found in the urine in about 10% of cases.

56–60. The answers are: 56-B, 57-E, 58-C, 59-A, 60-D. [*Chapter 4 II A 2 d, B 2 a–c (1) (2); III B 1–4, C*] In the classical pathway of complement activation, circulating C3 binds to the C$\overline{4b2a}$ complex (C3 convertase) and is cleaved into two fragments, C3a and C3b.

In the alternative pathway of complement activation, the complex C3b,B is susceptible to enzymatic cleavage by factor D. The Ba fragment is released and the C$\overline{3b,Bb}$ complex becomes a C3 convertase. C3a, along with C5a and C4a, are anaphylotoxins which cause release of vasoactive amines from mast cells and basophils. Their biological activity is enzymatically destroyed by anaphylatoxin inactivator.

Bb, a factor generated by the alternative but not the classical pathway of complement activation, activates macrophages and causes them to adhere to and spread on cell surfaces. It is a component of the C$\overline{3b,Bb}$ complex (C3 convertase), and its dissociation from the complex is slowed by properdin. Assembly of the membrane attack complex is triggered by cleavage of C5.

The larger cleavage product, C5b, forms a trimolecular complex with C6 and C7. The membrane-bound C5b67 complex then binds C8 and C9. The C5b6789 complexes induce formation of hollow cylinders in the cell membrane leading ultimately to osmotic lysis of the cell.

Natural Immunity

I. INTRODUCTION

A. Natural immunity (resistance) is the summation of all the naturally occurring defense mechanisms that protect an individual from infectious diseases. These physiologic mechanisms are present throughout the animal kingdom as inherent, or **innate**, qualities of the species. **They do not exhibit specificity** (i.e., they are not dependent on specific recognition of a foreign material). A single defense barrier will afford protection against many different potential pathogens.

B. Acquired immunity is a **specific immunologic response** that occurs following exposure to a particular infectious agent, either deliberate (vaccination) or accidental (infection). Increased resistance to that particular agent usually occurs as a result of the production of antibodies or sensitized lymphocytes specific for that microbe.

1. This immunity may be acquired by **natural** or **artificial** processes. For example, convalescent immunity that occurs when a person recovers from an infection is a naturally acquired immunity, whereas vaccination for the induction of an immune state is an artificial process. Similarly, placental passage of antibody is natural, whereas injection of gamma globulin is artificial.

2. Specific immunologic responses are mediated by two interrelated and interdependent mechanisms.

a. Humoral immunity primarily involves **bursa or bone marrow-derived (B) lymphocytes**, or **B cells**. These cells express specific **immunoglobulin** on their surface. When this interacts with its homologous antigen, the B cell is triggered to differentiate into a **plasma cell**, which excretes vast quantities of immunoglobulin of the same specificity. These proteins in the plasma fraction of the blood comprise the humoral component of the immune system.

b. Cell-mediated (cellular) immunity primarily involves **thymus-derived (T) lymphocytes**, or **T cells**. These T cells express on their surface a receptor molecule that is similar to an immunoglobulin and is specific for a particular antigen. Contact with the latter molecule stimulates proliferation and differentiation of the T cells. Cell-mediated immunity is the end product of this developmental process and is expressed in the peripheral blood and lymphoid tissues throughout the body (see Chapter 5).

C. Nonspecific immunity is innate; **specific immunity** is developed as a result of experiences with individual pathogens. Examples of the two types of resistance mechanisms are presented in Table 1-1.

Table 1-1. Resistance Mechanisms

Type of Resistance	Examples
Nonspecific	Mucous membranes
	Phagocytic cells
	Enzymes in secretions
	Interferon
Specific	
Naturally acquired	Placental transfer of antibody (passive)
	Recovery from disease (active)
Artificially acquired	Administration of antitoxin (passive)
	Vaccination (active)

II. DETERMINANTS OF NATURAL RESISTANCE

A. Mechanical barriers and physiologic factors contribute to natural immunity by inhibiting attachment and penetration of infectious agents.

1. **Intact skin** is the first line of defense against infection. Consisting of the keratinized outer layer of dead cells and the successive layers of epidermis, undamaged skin is virtually impenetrable to all but a few organisms.

2. **Mucous coating** of epithelial and mucosal cells prevents contact between many pathogens and areas that are not covered by skin. Microorganisms and other particles are trapped in the viscous mucus and removed by other mechanisms.

3. **Shedding of cells** that carry microbes provides a mechanical cleansing action. Saliva, tears, perspiration, urine, and other body fluids assist in flushing microbes.

4. **The beating of cilia** on the epithelial cells in the respiratory tract removes contaminating microorganisms that become trapped in the mucus. Injury to this mechanism can be caused by smoking and alcoholism.

5. **Coughing** dislodges and expels the mucous blanket. Other physiologic functions, such as **sneezing** and **vomiting** as well as **diarrhea**, also eliminate pathogenic organisms.

6. Other physiologic factors also contribute to natural immunity.
   a. **Body temperature.** Many organisms do not infect humans because they grow poorly at 37°C.
   b. **Oxygen tension**, especially high in the lungs, inhibits growth of anaerobes.
   c. **Age.** Persons who are very young (aged 3 years or younger) or very old (aged 75 or older) are much more susceptible to infection due to their suboptimal immune responsiveness.
   d. **Hormonal balance** affects the host immune response. An increase in corticosteroids, for example, decreases the inflammatory response and lowers resistance to infection. Thus, persons receiving cortisone for control of autoimmune disease or graft rejection events have a heightened susceptibility to infectious agents.

B. Chemical and biochemical inhibitors of infection, found in body secretions, provide a natural defense against microorganisms that invade the body.

1. **Sebaceous gland secretions** contain antimicrobial factors (e.g., fatty acids and low pH). Most bacteria and many viral and fungal agents are susceptible to low concentrations of organic acids.

2. **Tears** contain the enzyme **lysozyme**, which lyses bacteria on contact via destruction of the cell wall. In particular, lysozyme is effective against gram-positive bacteria.

3. **The acid pH** found in most physiologic secretions prevents colonization by microorganisms. Urine and vaginal secretions, as well as the hydrochloric acid in stomach secretions, maintain acidic microenvironments. These environments kill most pathogenic microbes, while promoting the growth of nonpathogenic bacteria (e.g., lactobacilli).

C. Phagocytosis. Immunologic barriers to infection are present as humoral and cell-mediated responses, which usually work together to neutralize toxic materials or destroy pathogenic microorganisms. Humoral responses are primarily specific (i.e., involving **antibody development**), but can also be nonspecific [e.g., via **complement system activation** (see Chapter 4)]. While cell-mediated responses can be specific (e.g., involving T cells), they may also be nonspecific and involve **phagocytic cells**.

1. **Phagocytic cells.** Two groups of cells are responsible for **phagocytosis**, the process by which an ingested material is destroyed.
   a. **Neutrophils** circulate in the blood and migrate quickly in response to local invasion by microorganisms.
   b. **Monocytes** are derived from bone marrow stem cells and circulate in the blood. They migrate to the tissues, where they differentiate into **macrophages**, which reside in all body tissues (e.g., Kupffer cells of the liver).

2. **Characteristic phagocytic processes.** While neutrophils, monocytes, and macrophages are not the only cells that phagocytize, they are the most important. They share the following characteristics.
   a. **Ameboid movement.** Cell migration occurs in and out of blood vessels, and throughout the tissues.
   b. **Chemotaxis.** Movement of cells or organisms toward objects occurs in response to chemi-

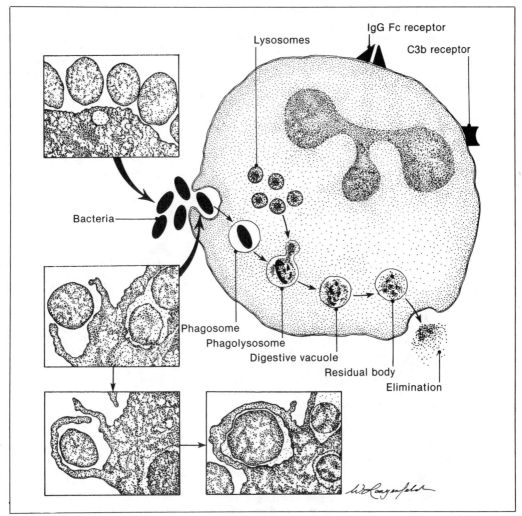

Figure 1-1. Composite schematic and corresponding electron microscopic representation of the process of phagocytosis. The illustration of an electron microscopic view demonstrates the phagocytosis of mycoplasma by macrophages following the addition of antimycoplasma antibody.

cal agents called **chemotaxins** (e.g., tissue components such as leukotriene, and activated intermediates of the fibrinolysis, kallikrein, and complement systems). When cells emigrate from capillaries, the process is called **diapedesis**.

  c. Phagocytosis. Once a particle is close enough to the target, the cells engulf it. A **phagocytic vacuole**, or **phagosome**, is formed by the phagocyte when it engulfs the particle and surrounds it with a part of its cell membrane. The membrane enclosing the particle pinches off and moves into the cytoplasm of the cell, where **lysosomes**, or membrane-bound bags of enzymes, fuse with the phagosome to form a **phagocytic lysosome**, or **phagolysosome** (Fig. 1-1).

  d. Cytopepsis* is the digestion of engulfed material inside the phagolysosome. The contents of the lysosome granules are important in breaking down ingested material and in killing microorganisms.

  (1) Lysosomal granules are of two types.

  (a) Primary granules, which comprise 33% of all granules, are also called **azurophilic granules**, so-named for their dark blue staining properties with Wright's stain. They contain many hydrolytic enzymes, myeloperoxidase, lysozyme, and arginine-rich basic (cationic) proteins.

---

*Term developed by the author.

    (b) **Secondary or specific granules**, which comprise 67% of all granules, contain alkaline phosphatase, lactoferrin, and lysozyme. Secondary granules release their contents into the phagosome first, usually before the vacuole has completely pinched off, so that the contents of secondary granules are partially expelled into the interstitial space, which is referred to as **exocytosis** (also called **regurgitation**). When this process is accelerated and primary granule contents are also released into the extracellular space, inflammation and tissue destruction can occur.

  (2) The contents of lysosomal granules include two mechanisms for destroying foreign particles.

    (a) Certain proteins kill microorganisms by **oxygen-independent mechanisms**, including:

      (i) Proteinases (hydrolytic enzymes)

      (ii) Cationic proteins [not enzymes, but basic peptides containing large amounts of arginine in polypeptide form that are highly antimicrobial (e.g., nuclear histones)]

      (iii) Lysozyme (a mucopeptidase that attacks bacterial cell walls) (see D 2 g)

      (iv) Lactoferrin (an iron-binding protein) (see D 2 e)

    (b) Other microbicidal compounds are generated by **oxygen-dependent mechanisms**, including:

      (i) Myeloperoxidase (catalyzes toxic peroxidation of a variety of microorganisms)

      (ii) Hydrogen peroxide (reactive oxidizing agent that kills microbes)

      (iii) Superoxide anion (molecular oxygen that has picked up an extra electron)

      (iv) Singlet oxygen (oxygen in which one of the electrons has moved to an orbit of higher energy)

      (v) Hydroxyl radical (a highly unstable oxidizing agent that reacts with most organic molecules it encounters)

  e. Secreted products. In addition to the intracellular destruction of foreign particles, phagocytic cells (specifically **macrophages**) also secrete many compounds that have a protective effect in the body. Among these are:

    (1) Factors that influence cell differentiation (e.g., colony-stimulating factor)

    (2) Cytotoxic factors (e.g., tumor necrosis factor)

    (3) Hydrolytic enzymes

    (4) Endogenous pyrogen (interleukin-1)

    (5) Complement components

    (6) Alpha interferon

3. Metabolic events during phagocytosis

  a. Metabolic events during phagocytosis are accompanied by a **respiratory burst** by the cell that involves the following:

    (1) An increase in **oxygen consumption**

    (2) Stimulation of **hexose monophosphate (HMP) shunt activity**

    (3) An increase in production of **hydrogen peroxide**

    (4) **Superoxide anion** production and **singlet oxygen** production

      (a) Superoxide anion is extremely toxic to bacteria and tissue, but it is very unstable and is quickly converted to hydrogen peroxide by the enzyme **superoxide dismutase**, which is still toxic to bacteria but is not as potent. The hydrogen peroxide is broken down by the enzyme, **catalase**.

      (b) A flaw in the formation of superoxide anion and eventually hydrogen peroxide is found in the neutrophils of persons suffering from **chronic granulomatous disease (CGD)**.

  b. The oxygen-dependent agents can combine and act synergistically; for example,

Myeloperoxidase + Hydrogen peroxide + Halide (I^- or Cl^-) → Hypochlorite

Hypochlorite is more antimicrobial than the three components alone. There are several mechanisms whereby such an activated halide could damage microorganisms (e.g., **halogenation of the bacterial cell wall** or decarboxylation of amino acids with the resultant production of **toxic aldehydes**).

4. Tests for measuring phagocytic function

  a. Chemotaxis. Phagocytic cells will migrate toward a chemotactic stimulus such as **endotoxin** or the complement split products, **C5a** and **C5b67**. If this movement occurs through an agar menstrum or across a 5 μ-pore size membrane, it can be measured and the chemotactic ability of the cells assessed.

  b. Phagocytosis. Cells can be incubated with bacteria or other engulfable materials (e.g., latex or polystyrene particles) for 1–2 hours, then stained and examined for uptake of the foreign bodies.

    c. Nitroblue tetrazolium reduction. This yellow water-soluble dye converts to a purple water-insoluble intracellular compound called **formazan** when phagocytizing neutrophils produce hydrogen peroxide and superoxide anion during the phagocytic process (see Chapter 8 IV A 1).

    d. Chemiluminescence. Singlet oxygen produces a small amount of light when its electron returns to its own original orbit. If normal levels of singlet oxygen are being produced, the light produced can be measured as chemiluminescence.

    e. Microbicidal activity. Intracellular killing by phagocytic cells can be measured by direct plate counting of mixtures of microorganisms and cells, or the viability of the engulfed microbes can be determined by the use of supravital stains such as acridine orange.

5. Opsonization. Phagocytosis can occur in a very simple system. For example, if neutrophils, saline, and bacteria are combined, phagocytosis will occur. Phagocytosis can be remarkably enhanced in the presence of blood serum or plasma, however, because of **opsonization**, which is the process of enhancing phagocytosis via the presence of **opsonins** (i.e., substances that promote phagocytosis). Opsonins found in serum include the following.

    a. The C3b split product of the complement cascade is the most important complement-derived opsonin; C4b and C5b are much less active in this process (see Chapter 4, section II A 2 d). Phagocytic cells possess a membrane receptor for C3b; thus, bacteria and other foreign materials that have this molecule on their surface will have an enhanced interaction with the phagocyte.

    b. C5a and **C5b67** are chemotactic factors that also aid in the clearance of foreign materials from the body.

    c. Antibodies are part of a group of proteins called **immunoglobulins (Ig)** [see Chapter 3]. Phagocytic cells also have a receptor for the Fc portion of IgG molecules, thus enhancing the strength of interaction between the cell and the antibody-coated or antibody-opsonized particle that is being engulfed. IgG1 and IgG3 are the most active in this process. There is a suggestion that IgA may also be an opsonin for phagocytosis by neutrophils and macrophages.

    d. Fibronectin is a glycoprotein that opsonizes and also acts like glue to cause neutrophils and their targets to stick together.

    e. Leukotrienes are derivatives of arachidonic acid; there are several kinds of leukotrienes, and they do not all act like opsonins. Leukotriene LTBy is chemotactic.

    f. Tuftsin is a tetrapeptide split product of IgG that stimulates chemotactic and phagocytic activities.

D. Humoral factors with antimicrobial activity

1. Normal serum can kill and lyse gram-negative bacteria. This property is probably due to normal antibody and complement, both present in normal serum. The activity is destroyed by heating at 56°C for 30 minutes, due to the inactivation of complement.

    a. Bacteriolysis occurs due to the lytic action of antibody-activated complement on the outer lipopolysaccharide layer of the cell wall.

    b. A bacterial cell wall contains two layers: an outer layer containing **lipopolysaccharide** and an inner layer of **mucopeptide (peptidoglycan).** The antibody and complement disrupt the lipopolysaccharide layer of the cell wall. Complement becomes an esterase, which provides for the majority of this enzymatic activity. Once the lipopolysaccharide layer is weakened, **lysozyme** (a mucopeptidase) present in serum can enter and destroy the mucopeptide layer. The end result is the destruction of the bacterial cell target.

2. Nonantibody factors contributing to natural immunity include the following.

    a. Chemotactic factors. Phagocytes are attracted primarily to complement split products, C5a and the trimolecular complex C5b67.

    b. Properdin is a protein different from normal antibody and complement but believed to work in conjunction with the two (plus magnesium ions) to effect bactericidal action. It is involved in complement activation by the **alternate pathway** (see Chapter 4, section II B).

    c. Beta lysin is an antibacterial protein released from blood platelets when they rupture, as in clot formation. It is active primarily against gram-positive bacteria.

    d. Interferons are proteins produced by virally infected cells, and they protect other cells in the area. Interferons induce neighboring cells to produce antiviral proteins that interfere with the translation of viral messenger RNA (mRNA).

        (1) Types of interferons include the following.

            (a) Alpha interferon—secreted by leukocytes—is induced by viruses or synthetic polynucleotides.

            (b) Beta interferon—secreted by fibroblasts—is induced by viruses or synthetic polynucleotides.

            (c) Gamma interferon—also called **immune interferon**—is secreted by lymphocytes following stimulation with specific antigen to which the lymphocyte has been sensitized.

    (2) Interferon activates cellular genes to produce antiviral proteins, which block viral translation by two enzyme-mediated processes.

        (a) Protein kinase transfers a phosphate group from adenosine triphosphate (ATP) to an initiation factor required for protein synthesis. When phosphorylated, the factor does not function properly and viral protein synthesis is inhibited.

        (b) Oligonucleotide polymerase synthesizes adenine trinucleotide, which activates an endonuclease in the cell to cleave mRNAs to prevent viral replication.

    (3) Interferon also enhances T-cell activity, activates macrophages, and increases the cytotoxic action of **natural killer (NK) cells**.

  e. Lactoferrin is an iron-binding protein that competes with bacteria for that essential metabolite. Transferrin, a serum beta globulin that is contained in phagocytes, acts similarly in binding and removing iron.

  f. Lactoperoxidase is found in saliva and milk. Its mechanism of action is similar to that of myeloperoxidase which serves microbicidal role.

  g. Lysozyme hydrolyzes the mucopeptide layer of the cell wall of many different bacteria. It is present in tears, saliva, nasal secretions, and other body fluids.

E. Lymphocytic cells contributing to natural immunity. A group of lymphocytic cells, which occur naturally in the body, express cytotoxicity against a variety of targets in the absence of any previous exposure to the foreign materials.

  1. NK cells are large granular lymphocytes that appear to have an immune surveillance function.

    a. They are spontaneous in their presence in the body and are cytotoxic for tumor cells and virally infected autologous cells.

    b. NK cells bear a small amount of the T-cell membrane marker, **Thy-1**, but lack most of the other membrane characteristics of T cells, although they are weakly reactive with sheep red blood cells (SRBCs), forming rosettes at 4°C but not at 29°C.

    c. NK cells have a membrane receptor for the **Fc portion of antibody** (see Chapter 3, section II E 1 b) but will kill targets in the absence of antibody.

    d. Their target range is broad, and they are not restricted by the **major histocompatibility complex (MHC)** [see Chapter 12, section II B 1 d] (i.e., NK cells do not require matching of MHC molecules between effector and target cells).

    e. NK cells release numerous cytokines during their interaction with the target cells, including **alpha and gamma interferons**, **interleukins-1 and -2**, **B-cell growth factor**, and **lymphotoxin**.

    f. Cytotoxic activity can be significantly enhanced by exposure to interleukin-2 and the interferons.

  2. Antibody-dependent cytotoxic cells can kill targets without the participation of complement.

    a. Killer (K) cells have cytotoxic activity with target cells coated with specific antibody in an **antibody-dependent cellular cytotoxic (ADCC) reaction**. These cells are present prior to antigenic exposure to the target. K cells bear receptors for the Fc portion of IgG molecules, and this is the mechanism of target recognition and interaction.

    b. ADCC is thought to play a role in antitumor and antigraft immunity and may be involved in antiviral protection as well.

    c. In addition to K cells, macrophages and neutrophils also participate in ADCC.

  3. The **lymphokine activated killer (LAK) cell** is another naturally occurring cytotoxic cell. It is a quiescent lymphocyte that is induced into an active cytotoxic state by the lymphokine interleukin-2. It is similar in many ways to the NK cell but has an even broader target cell range.

III. SIGNIFICANCE OF NATURAL IMMUNITY SYSTEMS. When there is an imbalance in any of the systems involved in natural immunity, the host has trouble with **"opportunistic" bacteria**. When the defenses of the host are diminished, these opportunists, which are organisms not ordinarily considered pathogenic, can become pathogenic and produce disease.

A. The oral cavity is most certainly the primary portal of entry for most microorganisms and will be discussed briefly to exemplify the various mechanisms serving to protect the host from infectious disease. Many factors seem to be involved in oral defense against microorganisms. These can be broadly grouped into three categories.

  1. Anatomic and physiologic barriers such as epithelium, flow of saliva, and anatomy of the teeth

  2. Cellular defenses such as normal phagocytosis by leukocytes and macrophages

3. Humoral immunity as the result of the antibody content of saliva

B. The oral mucosa is composed of stratified squamous epithelium, which forms an important mechanical barrier to infection. It depends primarily on two mechanisms for protection.

1. Constant desquamation rids the mouth of bacteria adherent to the epithelial cells.

2. The degree of keratinization influences the efficiency of the barrier.
   a. A **balance** is achieved by these two features. The hard palate and gingiva are completely keratinized; the gingival pocket epithelium is not keratinized and is composed of a very few cell layers, so it offers a rather weak barrier for oral defense. It does contribute to self-cleansing, however, by the continuous outward migration of cells due to constant desquamation.
   b. Close contact between pocket epithelium and tooth surfaces decreases the possibility of penetration by microorganisms.

C. Saliva is a mucous coating in the oral cavity that traps microorganisms and may have antibacterial properties. The flow of saliva backward to the throat, where it is swallowed, also helps to clear the oral cavity of organisms.

1. A slow flow rate favors caries and **parotitis**, or inflammation of the parotid glands.
   a. A pH of 4.0–5.5 favors the growth of **aciduric**, **acidogenic** microorganisms; therefore, a higher pH is better for the prevention of caries.
   b. Antibodies are contained in parotid fluid and saliva. They are synthesized by plasma cells in lymphoid tissues of the oral cavity.

2. Immunoglobulin A (IgA) predominates in saliva (see Chapter 3, section III B), with some IgG and IgM, perhaps from **gingival pocket fluid**.
   a. Gingival fluid contains lysozyme, antibodies, and other proteins comparable to serum.
   b. The fluid flows outward and has a fibrinolytic system that prevents clot formation, which would occlude the crevice.

STUDY QUESTIONS

Directions: Each question below contains five suggested answers. Choose the **one best** response to each question.

1. Innate immunity can be defined as

(A) the immunity resulting from vaccination
(B) the resistance to infectious diseases acquired via subclinical infections
(C) the naturally occurring defense mechanisms that provide protection from infectious agents
(D) the protection acquired due to placental passage of maternal antibodies
(E) the resistance dependent on specific recognition of infectious diseases

2. The process by which normal serum enhances phagocytosis is called

(A) chemotaxis
(B) opsonization
(C) proteolysis
(D) bacteriolysis
(E) exocytosis

3. Interferons can be described as

(A) interfering directly with translation of viral mRNA
(B) blocking the penetration of viruses into susceptible cells
(C) inducing the production of antiviral proteins that interfere with translation of viral RNA
(D) interfering with viral adsorption onto the cell membrane
(E) inducing host cell RNAse that hydrolyzes the viral genome

Directions: Each question below contains four suggested answers of which **one or more** is correct. Choose the answer

> A   if **1, 2, and 3** are correct
> B   if **1 and 3** are correct
> C   if **2 and 4** are correct
> D   if **4** is correct
> E   if **1, 2, 3, and 4** are correct

4. The respiratory system is protected from microorganisms by

(1) ciliary movement of the mucous blanket upward to the oropharynx
(2) body temperature regulation at 37°C
(3) expulsion of mucus-entrapped microbes by the cough reflex
(4) low oxygen tension, which slows growth of pathogenic bacteria

5. Antimicrobial products of the myeloperoxidase system include

(1) superoxide anions
(2) toxic aldehydes
(3) hypochlorite
(4) hydrogen peroxide

6. The lysosomal granules in the cytoplasm of phagocytic cells contain

(1) proteinases
(2) cationic proteins
(3) mucopeptidase
(4) lactoferrin

7. Macrophages secrete many antimicrobial factors, including

(1) tumor necrosis factor
(2) interleukin-1
(3) complement
(4) alpha interferon

C3b A67
C5 leukotriene

8. Opsonins found in serum include

(1) C3b
(2) antibody
(3) fibronectin
(4) tuftsin

E

9. Lymphocytic cells contributing to native immunity include

(1) natural killer (NK) cells
A (2) killer (K) cells
(3) lymphokine activated killer (LAK) cells
(4) neutrophils

ANSWERS AND EXPLANATIONS

1. The answer is C. (*I A, B 1, 2*) Innate immunity is a complex system of all naturally occurring defense mechanisms that protect individuals from infectious disease. While innate, or natural, resistance is a nonspecific immunity, acquired resistance is a specific immunologic response that occurs following deliberate exposure (e.g., a vaccination) or accidental exposure (e.g., infection) to a foreign agent. Acquired immunity can be actively acquired by natural processes, such as that induced by subclinical infections, or passively acquired, such as the transplacental passage of antibody to the human fetus.

2. The answer is B. (*II C 5*) Opsonization is the process whereby phagocytosis is enhanced. Chemotaxis is the direct movement of cells either toward (positive) or away from (negative) stimuli. Proteolysis is the breakup of protein molecules, and bacteriolysis is the dissolution of bacterial cells, which result from enzymatic attack of the cell wall or through the action of antibiotics on cell wall synthesis. These latter two events would occur during the cytopeptic process that follows the formation of the phagolysosome. Exocytosis, also called regurgitation, occurs when the contents of the lysosomal granules are expelled into the extracellular environment prior to closure of the vacuole.

3. The answer is C. (*II D 2 d*) There are no antiviral compounds known today that interfere *directly* with translation of viral mRNA, although interferon does activate a cellular nuclease that degrades it. Interferon also induces the host cell to produce other RNA and protein inhibitors. Certain antiviral chemotherapeutics, such as amantadine, inhibit viral adsorption and/or penetration of host cells. Antibody is most effective in blocking viral adsorption onto a cell membrane. Interferon induces the cell to produce an oligonucleotide polymerase which synthesizes adenine trinucleotide that activates an endonuclease in the cell.

4. The answer is A (1, 2, 3). (*II A 2, 4, 5, 6 b*) Mucus entraps inhaled microorganisms. These are removed from the respiratory tract via the mucous blanket escalator, which delivers them to the esophagus, where they are swallowed or expelled from the body by the cough reflex. Body temperature contributes to natural resistance, since many organisms grow poorly at 37°C. The oxygen tension in the lungs is high, thus inhibiting the growth of anaerobes; whereas low oxygen tension favors the growth of many human pathogens.

5. The answer is E (all). (*II C 3 a, b*) In addition to toxic aldehydes and superoxide anions, antimicrobial products of the myeloperoxidase system include singlet oxygen, hydrogen peroxide, and myeloperoxidase itself, working in concert with halide ions to produce hypochlorite.

6. The answer is E (all). [*II C 2 d (2) (a) (i)–(iv)*] Lysosomal granules contain many proteins that kill via oxygen-independent means, such as proteinases, cationic proteins, mucopeptidase, and lactoferrin. Other microbicidal compounds are generated by oxygen-dependent mechanisms, including hydrogen peroxide, superoxide anion, and singlet oxygen. The low pH attained intracellularly is also antimicrobial.

7. The answer is E (all). [*II C 2 e (1)–(6)*] Macrophages secrete tumor necrosis factor, interleukin-1, complement, and alpha interferon, as well as many other substances. Enzymes such as cathepsins and phosphatases are released, as are compounds, such as colony-stimulating factor, which influence cell differentiation. These substances are called monokines because they are the products of mononuclear cells, either blood monocytes or tissue macrophages.

8. The answer is E (all). (*II C 5 a, c, d, f*) Opsonization is a process, the end result of which is an enhancement of phagocytosis. C3b, antibody, fibronectin, and tuftsin enhance the interaction of the phagocytic cell with the particle to be engulfed. Other enhancers of phagocytosis are the chemotactic factors C5a and C5b67, which attract phagocytes to areas of inflammation. Leukotrienes (lipoxygenase metabolites of arachidonic acid) may also increase the rate of phagocytosis due to their vasodilatory effect, which would increase the blood flow in the area.

9. The answer is A (1, 2, 3). (*II E 1–3*) Native immunity is the resistance to disease that a person has without prior exposure to the agent in question. Natural killer (NK) and lymphokine activated killer (LAK) cells are active in tumor and graft rejection and in recovery from infections caused by intracellular parasites such as viruses. Killer (K) cells are involved in antibody-dependent cellular cytotoxic (ADCC) reactions. Neutrophils are important scavenger cells of the body and are a major part of native immunity; however, they are from the granulocytic series, not the lymphocytic series, of blood cells.

2
Immunogenicity and Antigens

I. DEFINITIONS

A. Antigens. An antigen must possess two properties.

    1. Immunogenicity is the inherent ability of a substance (**immunogen**) to induce a specific immune response, resulting in the formation of antibodies or immune lymphocytes.

    2. Specific reactivity, or **antigenicity**, is the property of a substance (**antigen**) that causes it to react specifically with the antibody or cell that it caused to be produced.

        a. The property of antigenicity is extremely important. It is probably the most specific reaction known in biology.

        b. Immunogenic substances are always antigenic, whereas **antigens are not necessarily immunogenic**.

B. Haptens are partial antigens that are antigenic but not immunogenic (e.g., dinitrophenol and penicillin).

    1. Haptens cannot cause the production of immune lymphocytes or antibodies, but they can react.

    2. Haptens are usually smaller molecules, which are too small to be considered immunogens. If they are coupled to a larger **carrier molecule**, however, they become endowed with immunogenicity. Carrier molecules may be albumins, globulins, or synthetic polypeptides.

C. Determinant groups, or **epitopes**, are sites either on or within the antigen with which the antibodies react.

    1. Epitopes determine the specificity of the molecule and are what induce the antibody response. Antibodies are specific for the epitopes, which are very small (e.g., just four or five amino acid or monosaccharide residues).

    2. Haptens and epitopes are similar, but while a hapten is artificially added to a molecule, an epitope is an integral part of the native molecule.

    3. Antigens are multivalent; that is, they may have hundreds of epitopes, some specifying antibody "A," others antibody "B," and so forth. The valence of the antigen will be equal to the total number of epitopes the antigen possesses.

    4. Antigen molecules can be artificially manipulated by adding or taking away epitopes. Every time one is changed, antigenicity is altered.

        a. New antigens are produced by altering these epitopes. This can be done by conjugating haptens to the molecule.

        b. A classic example in human medicine is the **allergic response** of some persons to penicillin. A derivative of penicillin, **penicilloic acid**, acting as a hapten, can couple with body protein and elicit an immune response that can be harmful, even life threatening, thus excluding this antibiotic from use in certain individuals.

    5. The epitopes on an antigen can be **linear** (e.g, within the amino acid sequence of the molecule) or **conformational** (e.g., containing amino acids that appear in the same area on the surface of the protein but not adjacent in the peptide chain). Denaturation or hydrolysis of the protein will almost always destroy conformational epitopes (see Fig. 2-1).

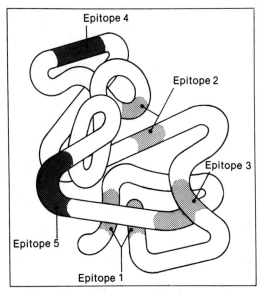

Epitope 4

Epitope 2

Epitope 3

Epitope 5

Epitope 1

Figure 2-1. Model of epitopes on lysozyme. The *shaded areas* are the specific epitopes. They are composed of chain segments that are either linear (epitopes 4 and 5) or conformational (epitopes 1–3). (Adapted from Klein J: Immunology: The Science of Self–Nonself Discrimination. New York, John Wiley & Sons, 1982, p 356.)

II. PROPERTIES OF IMMUNOGENICITY. The degree of immunogenicity of a molecule is influenced by several factors. The relationship can be expressed algebraically by the following formula:

Immunogenicity = (foreignness) (chemical complexity) (molecular size).

The interaction of the factors is not simply additive, as materials that have no foreignness (F = 0) are **nonantigenic**, and the immunogenicity of identical molecules can be greatly enhanced by increases in molecular size via chemical or heat aggregation.

A. Foreignness. An antigen must be foreign or alien to the host to which it is administered.

   1. Autologous antigens are found within the same individual; that is, it is not foreign. A skin graft from an individual's thigh to his own back is an **autograft**.

   2. Syngeneic antigens are found in individuals of an inbred strain (or between identical twins) who are, then, genetically identical. A graft between members of an inbred strain is a syngeneic graft or an **isograft**.

   3. Allogeneic or **homologous** antigens are found within the same species but between different individuals. For example, a kidney transplant from mother to daughter is called a **homograft** or **allograft. Isoantigens (alloantigens)** occur in certain members of the species and not in others. This term is used to designate the A and B blood group antigens.

   4. Xenogeneic or **heterologous** antigens are found across species boundaries. For example, a transplant of monkey kidneys to humans is called a **xenograft**. The greater the phylogenetic difference, the more foreign something becomes.
      a. Heterogenetic (heterophil) antigens are those which occur in different species. The spirochete that causes syphilis has a heterogenetic antigen similar to a hapten called **cardiolipin** found in beef heart muscle.
      b. The heterophile antigen has a practical application as it forms the basis of diagnostic tests for syphilis. The principle of **heterophil antibody response** is also the basis of a test used in the diagnosis of infectious mononucleosis caused by the Epstein-Barr herpesvirus, as most of these patients have present in their serum an antibody that reacts with sheep red blood cells (SRBCs). Rickettsial infections induce in the affected person the agglutination of certain strains of *Proteus Vulgaris* (i.e., OX-19, OX-2, and OX-K), which is another heterophilic immune response termed the **Weil-Felix reaction**.

   5. Sequestered antigens. Antibodies are not ordinarily made to autologous brain or cornea protein because these substances do not come in contact with antibody-producing cells since they are inaccessible to antibody-forming tissues (i.e., they are "sequestered").
      a. The central nervous system is devoid of lymphatics, as is the cornea, which is also nonvascularized; both are required for an immune response. If sequestered antigens are released (i.e., if sequestered tissue is exposed to the antibody-producing lymphoreticular system), then an immune response may result.
      b. Experimental allergic encephalomyelitis can be produced in animals by injection of ho-

mologous or heterologous brain tissue in Freund's adjuvant [a mixture of killed bacteria and oil] (see Chapter 6, section IV A 1). The antigen is a **basic protein** in myelin.

6. **Tissue-specific antigens.** Various organs have in their makeup certain antigens common and unique to those organs.

   a. **Thyroid** has an organ-specific antigen. Any thyroid from any species contains this unique thyroid antigen, thyroglobulin.

   b. Another example is **basic protein**, which exists in brain tissue regardless of species, but does not exist in any other organ.

B. **Chemical complexity.** With the exception of pure lipids, most organic chemical groupings can be immunogens.

1. The majority of immunogens are **proteins**. Because they have the largest array of potential building blocks (**amino acids**), they are the strongest antigens. This diversity imparts epitopes of differing specificities to the molecule. The total immune response will be the sum of all the individual antibodies that are produced. Immunogenicity can also be enhanced by adding haptens (i.e., new determinant groups) to the molecule.

   a. **Bacterial and mammalian cells** are also strong immunogens, and present a vast array of different epitopes to the host.

   b. **Lipoproteins** are special types of protein immunogens that exist as part of many cell membranes.

2. **Polysaccharides.** Most polysaccharides are haptens or incomplete immunogens because they do not possess sufficient chemical diversity. In addition, they are usually rapidly degraded when injected; thus, they are not in contact with the immune apparatus long enough to induce a response. However, polysaccharides can be immunogens, occurring in two forms:

   a. **Pure polysaccharide substances** (e.g., pneumococcal capsule polysaccharides, which are responsible for the protective immune response to the pneumococcus)

   b. **Lipopolysaccharides**, which occur within the cell membranes of gram-negative bacteria (e.g., endotoxins)

3. The immunogenicity of **glycoproteins** is best illustrated by the blood group antigens A and B and the Rh antigens. The A and B substances are strong immunogens, and the immune response they induce is to the carbohydrate epitope of the molecule (see Chapter 12 II B 1; D 1).

4. **Polypeptide immunogens** include hormones (e.g., insulin and growth hormones) and synthetic compounds such as polylysine. These are usually weakly immunogenic.

5. **Nucleic acids** are considered to be nonimmunogenic; however, when single-stranded, they can act as immunogens. Nucleoproteins are stronger immunogens because the nucleic acid is coupled to protein. In patients with systemic lupus erythematosus, antibodies to nucleoproteins are produced.

6. **Lipids** (e.g., cardiolipin) are also nonimmunogenic, although a few can function as haptens.

C. **Molecular size.** Usually the larger the molecule, the better the immunogen, although there are exceptions.

1. As a general rule, molecules below 5000 daltons will not be immunogenic: Reasonable immune responses will be induced by molecules like serum albumin (40,000 daltons); gamma globulin (160,000) and hemocyanin (1,000,000) are excellent immunogens.

2. **Size** is important because of the following reasons.

   a. The number of epitopes increases proportionately with the size of the protein.

   b. Larger size means the molecule is going to be **phagocytized**. Antibodies to certain antigens are formed more rapidly if the antigen is first somehow **"processed" by a macrophage**. Soluble antigen is difficult or impossible to phagocytize and therefore is not immunogenic at times.

III. "GOOD" IMMUNOGENS

A. **The result of active immunization** is the production of protective antibodies directed at the virulence factors of the pathogen. There are four types of vaccines:

1. **Killed organisms** (e.g., typhoid bacilli)

2. **Attenuated or altered live agents** (e.g., Sabin polio virus)

3. Detoxified toxins (e.g., diphtheria and tetanus toxoids)

4. Artificially assembled microbial components (e.g., hepatitis B virus subunits)

B. Examples of good immunogens

1. All gram-negative, flagellated bacteria (e.g., *Salmonella typhi*) contain two types of antigens, to which the host organism makes different antibodies. The two antigens are:
   a. The "H" antigens, referring to the flagella
   b. The "O" antigens, referring to the body of the organism

2. Any bacterial cell is a good immunogen. Actually, hundreds of different antibodies are formed in response to the bacterial cell, but the only protective antibodies are those directed against the factors of the bacterial cell that gives it the ability to cause disease, (i.e., the bacterial cell's **virulence factors**). For example, the polysaccharides of the pneumococcal capsule must be neutralized if the virulence of the pneumococcus is to be overcome, since the capsule is antiphagocytic.

3. The same is true for **diphtheria** and **tetanus toxins**. Protection from them can be obtained if antibodies to these toxins are produced, since the toxins are what cause the diseases. Also **lipopolysaccharide** (endotoxin) is a major virulence factor for gram-negative bacteria, and antibody against this is needed for protection.

IV. CHEMICAL BASIS OF ANTIGEN SPECIFICITY

A. Haptens. The exquisite sensitivity of the immune response has been studied through the use of haptens. Haptens can be side chains of benzene rings, or substituted benzene rings, that are attached to protein molecules and, hence, rendered immunogenic. The immune response can then be mounted against both the carrier protein and the hapten. An illustration of the specificity of the immune response in relation to haptens is shown in Figure 2-2.

1. All of the **substituted groups are in the para-position**; however, the parasubstituted group is different in each case.

2. The immune response generated by any one of these **conjugated hapten groups** is completely cross-reactive against the others. Apparently, the host can recognize the para-position but not the substituent groups (as long as they remain chemically similar).

3. On the other hand, the host organism can distinguish between ortho-positions and para-positions, and the antibodies formed are not cross-reactive (Fig. 2-3).

B. Capsular antigens. A more clinically relevant example of this specificity can be demonstrated by considering the antibodies to the **capsular antigens** of the pneumococcus, one of the major causes of lobar pneumonia.

1. There are approximately 80+ different immunologic types of pneumococcus. An antibody of one type does not react with an antigen of another type. These capsular polysaccharides are structurally different, which accounts for their antigenic differences.

2. The type II pneumococcal capsule has in its structure only glucose in 1–4, 1–6 linkages. The antibody directed against pneumococcus type II is directed against this glucose polymer. This is known because these antibodies will react with glucose 1–4, 1–6 linkages regardless of where they are found (e.g., those found in glycogen). This is so specific that it can be used to determine if the 1–4, 1–6 linkage exists in unknown polysaccharides.

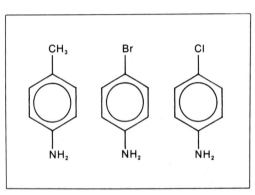

Figure 2-2. Examples of cross-reactive substituted benzene haptens. If a carboxyl group was in the para-position, the hapten would not react with antibody against the illustrated haptens.

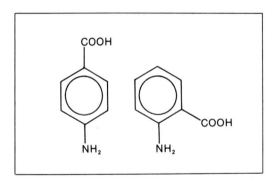

Figure 2-3. Examples of non-cross-reactive substituted benzene haptens. The change from para- to ortho-substitution produces a new specificity.

    C. Adjuvants. Nonspecific stimulation of the immune response can occur via **adjuvants** (see Chapter 6, section IV A). Adjuvants are substances that enhance the immunogenicity of molecules without altering their chemical composition. The mechanisms by which adjuvants exert their biological effects is uncertain. **Complete Freund's adjuvant**, a mixture of killed bacteria and oil, is a classic adjuvant that can enhance an immune response to an antigen.

V. FORCES OF ANTIGEN–ANTIBODY ATTRACTION. The **antigen–antibody complex** is not bound firmly together. It may even dissociate spontaneously; however, the equilibrium is far to the right. Various forces act to hold the complex together.

    A. Van der Waals forces are allowed to act due to spatial fit (Fig. 2-4). The forces act to hold antigen to antibody on the left; they do not act as well on the right.

    B. Coulombic forces (Fig. 2-5) are patterns of electrical charge on the molecule that are complementary. The electrostatic interactions tend to hold the molecules together.

        1. Antibody–antigen complexes are probably a mixture of both Van der Waals and coulombic forces.

        2. Another interesting fact involves the **accessibility of the epitope.** Using synthetic polypeptides, it has been shown that only those amino acids that are spatially accessible due to tertiary protein structure are able to be immunoreactive.

    C. Proteins can exist as **globular** or **fibrous** proteins or mixtures of the two, but the very **nature of the structure** is highly important. The ability of the antibody to bind to the antigenic sites can be affected by altering the tertiary structure. The antigenic sites would, then, no longer be spatially arranged such that antibody–antigen coupling could occur.

    D. Insulin molecules provide another illustration.

        1. Insulin has a molecular weight of approximately 6000, and is a weak antigen.

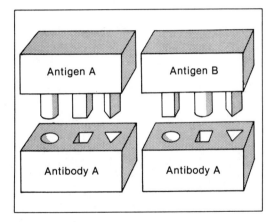

Figure 2-4. Influence of spatial fit on antigen–antibody reaction. Transposition of the *round* and *square pegs* diminishes the attraction between the two molecules.

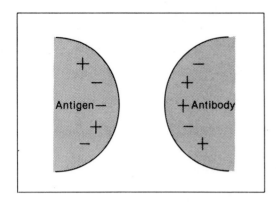

Figure 2-5. Pattern of electric charges on antigen and antibody influences interaction. As the pattern becomes more complementary, the force of attraction becomes proportionately stronger.

   2. It is composed of two chains, an **"A" chain** and a **"B" chain**.
      a. Antibody to either one of these chains can be produced by splitting the chains, purifying them, and injecting them into a foreign host that will produce antibodies to the particular chain injected.
      b. If these antibodies are injected back into the animal species that supplied the original insulin, this antibody will not react with intact insulin molecules. The explanation is that the tertiary structure of insulin must be such that the determinant groups on the molecule are accessible.

   3. Diabetics who need insulin for maintenance sometimes become **insulin tolerant**, and the insulin is no longer effective. Insulin varies among species by **three amino acid residues** sitting side-by-side on the A chain. Antibodies are formed to these three amino acids and inactivate the molecule.
      a. This is an example of the specificity of the immune response, especially in its ability to distinguish these small changes in such compounds as the various insulin molecules.
      b. The treatment for this antibody inactivation of the insulin is to **switch from beef to pork insulin**, where these three amino acids would be different.

E. Affinity and avidity

   1. The strength of the attraction between an epitope and the antigen combining site of the antibody molecule is referred to as the **affinity** of the reaction. Complexes of low affinity dissociate readily.

   2. A related term—**avidity**—refers to the strength of the interaction between complex antigens and the population of antibodies which they have induced. Avidity is influenced by the affinity of individual antibodies in the serum, the valence of the antigen, and the valence of the antibodies.

STUDY QUESTIONS

Directions: Each question below contains five suggested answers. Choose the **one best** response to each question.

1. An example of a sequestered antigen is

(A) penicillin
(B) diphtheria toxoid
(C) salmonella O antigens
(D) basic protein of myelin
(E) salmonella H antigens

2. Properties of haptens include

(A) immunogenicity and reactivity
(B) reactivity but no immunogenicity
(C) immunogenicity but no reactivity
(D) neither immunogenicity nor reactivity
(E) chemical complexity and macromolecular nature

3. A graft exchanged between brother and sister is termed

(A) xenograft
(B) isograft
(C) autograft
(D) allograft
(E) heterograft

4. An antigen that occurs irregularly in various tissues of different species is referred to as

(A) allogeneic
(B) syngeneic
(C) heterogenetic
(D) isogeneic
(E) sequestered

Directions: Each question below contains four suggested answers of which **one or more** is correct. Choose the answer

A   if **1, 2, and 3** are correct
B   if **1 and 3** are correct
C   if **2 and 4** are correct
D   if **4** is correct
E   if **1, 2, 3, and 4** are correct

5. Antigenic sites with which antibodies react are called

(1) immunogens
(2) determinant groups
(3) carriers
(4) epitopes

6. True statements concerning antigen epitopes include

(1) the same epitope will be expressed multiple times in the molecule
(2) the valence of the molecule will be equal to the total number of epitopes it has
(3) there will be several different types of epitopes in the molecule
(4) the valence of the molecule will be equal to the number of different antibody molecules that react with it in a precipitin assay

7. The degree of immunogenicity is influenced by

(1) molecular size
(2) degree of foreignness
(3) chemical composition
(4) presence of adjuvants

8. In order to be immunoreactive, an epitope must be

(1) part of a globular protein
(2) linear
(3) electronegative
(4) spatially accessible

9. Antigen–antibody complexes are not bound firmly together, but must be held together by

(1) Van der Waals forces
(2) proteins
(3) coulombic forces
(4) epitopes

ANSWERS AND EXPLANATIONS

1. The answer is D. (*II A 5 b*) The tissues of the central nervous system are not normally exposed to the immunologic apparatus of the host (i.e., they are "sequestered"). If they are exposed, an autoimmune disease could result. An immune response to the basic protein of the myelin sheath that surrounds neurons is thought to be involved in the autoimmune disease acute disseminated encephalomyelitis. Diphtheria toxoid and salmonella O and H antigens are exogenous antigens; penicillin is a hapten.

2. The answer is B. (*I B*) Haptens, by themselves, are unable to induce an immune response. They gain immunogenicity when they interact with a carrier molecule (usually an antigen itself). Haptens do possess the ability to react with their homologous antibody or lymphocyte, although this reactivity may not yield a visible manifestation. For example, simple haptens react with their homologous antibody, but the reaction cannot be visualized because no lattice structures are built-up; the hapten is monovalent. It will occupy both antigen-reactive sites on the antibody molecule, and will interfere with the antibody's precipitating capabilities. Simple hapten–antibody reactions are visualized, then, by the hapten's ability to block the precipitation of hapten–carrier complexes by the same antibody. Haptens are usually low molecular weight compounds and hence have a relatively simple chemical composition.

3. The answer is D. (*II A 3*) Grafts between members of the same species are termed allografts or homografts. Autografts occur when tissue is moved from one place to another on the same individual (e.g., skin transplants). Isografts occur between inbred animals and between identical twins, while xenografts cross species boundaries.

4. The answer is C. (*II A 4 a*) Heterogenetic, or heterophilic, antigens occur in widely separated places in the plant or animal kingdoms or both. The Forssman antigen, for example, is found on sheep red blood cells (SRBCs), guinea pig tissues, corn, and certain bacteria. Allogeneic antigens are present in some, but not all members of a species. Inbred animals are said to be antigenically syngeneic. Antigens that can generate an immune response in genetically different members of the same species, but not in the member carrying it, are called isogeneic.

5. The answer is C (2, 4). (*I C*) The area of an antigen with which an antibody reacts is one of the epitopes, or determinant groups, of that molecule. These are usually 4–6 residues (amino acids or monosaccharides) in size. These areas need not be linear within the molecule and could have proximity resulting from folding of the chain. The entire molecule is referred to as an immunogen. Carriers are molecules, usually proteins, which impart immunogenicity to haptens that are conjugated to them.

6. The answer is A (1, 2, 3). (*I C 3*) A single antigen will have multiple copies of several different epitopes. The larger the molecule, the greater will be the number of each. Increasing chemical complexity will increase the number of different epitopes as well. The valence of an antigen is the sum of all the epitopes possessed by that molecule, both spatially accessible and internal as well. Thus if the number of antibody molecules that react with an antigen is quantitated, the valence due to the internal epitope composition as well as the interference that will occur due to spatial competition for reaction sites will be underestimated.

7. The answer is E (all). (*II A–C, IV C*) The relative ability of a molecule to induce an immune response (i.e., immunogenicity) is influenced by molecular size, chemical nature, and degree of foreignness. These attributes are not simply additive, nor directly factorial, as a molecule of limited size may be highly immunogenic if it has sufficient complexity. Nonspecific stimulation of the immune response can occur via adjuvants, which can enhance immunogenicity without altering chemical composition.

8. The answer is D (4). (*I C 5*) An epitope must be on the outside of a molecule if the antibody is to be able to react with it, otherwise spatial interference would prevent the molecular interaction. Surface accessibility is not necessary for immunogenicity, however, as the cell or molecule may be broken down somewhat during phagocytic cell "processing," thus exposing internal epitope groups or antigens to the immunologic apparatus of the host.

9. The answer is A (1, 2, 3). (*V A, B, C*) Van der Waals and coulombic forces, as well as proteins, act to hold together antigen–antibody complexes. Van der Waals forces are allowed to act due to spatial fit. The electrostatic interactions of coulombic forces tend to hold the molecules together. The nature of the structure of globular or fibrous proteins can allow antibody to bind to antigenic sites, although particular changes to the tertiary structure of proteins could change the arrangement of antigenic sites and thus not allow antigen–antibody coupling.

3
Immunoglobulins

I. INTRODUCTION. Immunoglobulins (antibodies) are glycoproteins present in serum gamma globulins produced by B-lymphocytes (**B cells**) or plasma cells in response to exposure to antigen. They react specifically with that antigen in vivo or in vitro and are hence a part of the **adaptive immune response**, specifically, **humoral immunity**.

II. STRUCTURE

A. Basic unit. The basic structural unit (**monomer**) of immunoglobulin (Ig) molecules consists of **four polypeptide chains linked covalently by disulfide bonds** (Fig. 3-1). Polypeptide chains are composed of **amino acids** that are arranged in a sequence that identifies a given protein and distinguishes it from any other molecule. The four-chain structure is composed of two identical light (L) and two identical heavy (H) polypeptide chains.

1. **Light chains** have a molecular weight of approximately 23,000 and are composed of about 200 amino acids. Light chains are common to all immunoglobulin classes (**isotypes**) and are of two types—**kappa ($\varkappa$) or lambda (λ)**—based on their structural (antigenic) differences.
   a. The proportion of $\varkappa$ to λ chains in immunoglobulin molecules is about 2:1 in humans.
   b. A given immunoglobulin molecule may contain either identical $\varkappa$ or λ chains, but never both.

2. **Heavy chains** have a molecular weight approximately twice that of light chains (50,000–75,000) and twice the number of amino acids (about 400). Five antigenically distinct isotypes of heavy chains are recognized—gamma (γ), alpha (α), mu (μ), delta (δ), and epsilon (ϵ)—based on structural differences in the carboxy terminal portion of heavy chains.
   a. The heavy chain isotypes form the basis of five classes of immunoglobulin molecules—IgG (contains γ chain), IgA (contains α chain), IgM (contains μ chain), IgD (contains δ chain), IgE (contains ϵ chain) [see section III].
   b. Heavy chain classes are subdivided in subclasses of molecules. The subdivision is based on the greater degree of amino acid sequence relatedness shown by subclasses of the same class than by different classes.
   (1) Four known subclasses of the γ chain exist— γ_1, γ_2, γ_3, and γ_4—which yield IgG_1, IgG_2, IgG_3, and IgG_4.
   (2) Two subclasses of the α chain are known—α_1 and α_2—which yield IgA_1 and IgA_2.
   (3) Two subclasses of the μ chain are known—μ_1 and μ_2—which yield IgM_1 and IgM_2.
   (4) No subclasses of the δ and ϵ (i.e., IgD and IgE) have been demonstrated.

B. Disulfide bonds hold together the four polypeptide chains in normal immunoglobulin molecules, and are of two types.

1. **Interchain bonds** occur between heavy chains (H—H), heavy and light chains (H—L), and light chains (L—L).
   a. H—H bonds occur primarily in the **hinge region** (see section II F) and can vary in number from 1–15, depending on the class and subclass of the immunoglobulin molecule. These bonds also occur in the carboxy terminal portion of the heavy chain.
   b. H—L bonding occurs in most immunoglobulin molecules; an exception is IgA_2, which does not contain this bond. Only one disulfide bond attaches heavy and light chains.
   c. L—L bonds can occur under pathologic conditions (e.g., secretion of Bence-Jones protein).

2. **Intrachain bonds** are stronger than interchain bonds and occur within the individual chain type, with the number of bonds varying depending on the type (i.e., light chains have two, human γ, α and δ heavy chains have four, and human μ and ϵ heavy chains have five). The

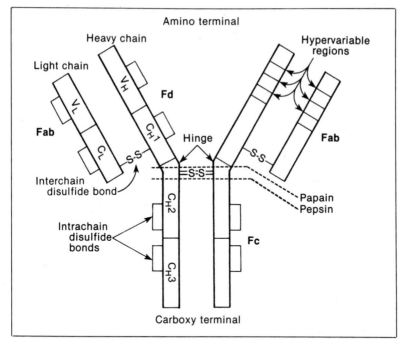

Figure 3-1. Basic unit (monomer) of IgG molecule consisting of four polypeptide chains linked covalently by disulfide bonds (S—S). *V* = variable region; *C* = constant region; *L* = light chain; *H* = heavy chain.

distribution of intrachain disulfide bonds forms the basis for division of each immunoglobulin into **domains** (see section II D).

C. Regions. Each heavy and light chain consists of two segments.

1. The **variable (V) region** shows a wide variation in amino acid sequence in the amino, or N, terminal portion of the molecule. The areas of high variability in the variable region of heavy (V_H) and light (V_L) chains are called **hypervariable regions ("hot spots")**.
   a. Hypervariable regions are most intimately involved in formation of the antigen-binding site.
   b. There are at least three hypervariable regions in both V_H and V_L regions (hv1—hv3).

2. The **constant (C) region** demonstrates an unvarying amino acid sequence in the carboxy, or C, terminal portion of the molecule, except for minor inherited differences.

D. Domains. Each immunoglobulin chain consists of a series of globular **homology regions** or **domains** enclosed by disulfide bonds.

1. Each heavy chain consists of four or five domains—one in the variable region (V_H) and three or four in the constant region (C_H1, C_H2, C_H3, and C_H4).
   a. The γ, α, and δ chains have four domains (one variable and three constant).
   b. The μ and ϵ chains have five domains (one variable and four constant).

2. Each light chain consists of two domains—one in the variable region (V_L) and one in the constant region (C_L).

3. Domains consist of about 110 amino acid residues. Peptide loops of 60–70 amino acid residues enclosed by intrachain disulfide bonds represent the central portion of each domain. The amino acid sequences of the loops show a high degree of homology.

E. Fragments. Proteolytic (peptide bond-splitting) enzymes are used to degrade immunoglobulin molecules into definable fragments to facilitate study of their structure. The primary agents used are **papain** and **pepsin**.

1. Treatment of the monomeric basic unit with the enzyme **papain** splits it into three fragments of approximately equal size at the hinge region (see section II F).

a. Two **Fab fragments** (**F**ragment-**a**ntigen **b**inding) each contain an entire light chain and the V_H and C_H1 domains of the heavy chain (or **Fd fragment**). These fragments can bind but cannot precipitate the antigen; therefore, they are **monovalent**, possessing only one combining site each. Fd, the amino terminal half of the heavy chain, has important biological function in that it provides the bulk of the antigen-binding capability of the Fab fragment.

b. One **Fc fragment** (**F**ragment **c**rystallizable) contains the carboxy terminal portion of the heavy chain. This portion of the molecule:
   (1) Binds complement
   (2) Contains carbohydrate
   (3) Dictates whether a given immunoglobulin can cross the placenta

2. Treatment of the immunoglobulin molecule with **pepsin** results in digestion of most of the Fc fragment, leaving one large fragment that consists of two Fab fragments joined by covalent bonds, termed the **F(ab')₂ fragment**. The F(ab')₂ fragment has two antigen-combining sites; thus, it is **bivalent**, possessing the ability to bind and precipitate an antigen.

F. **Hinge region.** The hinge region is the portion of the heavy chain between the C_H1 and C_H2 domains.

1. The region is considered as a separate domain because it is not homologous to any of the other known domains.

2. In this region, interchain disulfide bonds form between the arms of the Fab fragments, preventing them from folding and, thus, rendering this portion of the molecule highly susceptible to fragmentation by enzymatic attack.
   a. Papain cleaves the molecule on one side of the disulfide bonds, acting directly on the hinge region.
   b. Pepsin acts on the opposite side of the disulfide bonds, degrading the molecule just below the hinge region.

3. The hinge region is highly flexible and allows for movement of the Fab arms in relation to each other.

G. **S value.** Included among the properties of the immunoglobulins is their **sedimentation coefficient**, or **S value**, which expresses the behavior of a particle (protein) as determined via ultracentrifugation.

1. The behavior depends on the size and density of the particle, as well as the density and viscosity of the medium.

2. The sedimentation coefficient is expressed in **Svedberg units (S)**, with the S values of immunoglobulins ranging from 7S–19S.

III. **PROPERTIES AND ACTIVITY.** As indicated, immunoglobulins fall into five classes (isotypes) based on certain structural differences (Table 3-1). Each class also has certain unique biological and chemical properties.

A. **IgG** is the major immunoglobulin in normal human serum, accounting for approximately 75% of the total, most of which is IgG1, at a concentration of approximately 1200 mg/dl.

1. **Structure.** IgG is a monomer consisting of identical pairs of heavy and light chains linked by

Table 3-1. Structural Characteristics of Immunoglobulins

	IgG	IgA	IgM	IgD	IgE
H chain	γ	α	μ	δ	ϵ
H chain subclasses	$\gamma_1, \gamma_2, \gamma_3, \gamma_4$	α_1, α_2	μ_1, μ_2	–	–
Molecular weight	150,000	160,000–400,000	900,000	180,000	190,000
S value	7	7–18	19	7	8
Valence	2	2–8	10	2	2
J chain	–	+	+	–	–
Gm allotypes	+	–	–	–	–
Am allotypes	–	+	–	–	–
Km allotypes	+	+	+	+	+
L chain	$\varkappa, \lambda$	$\varkappa, \lambda$	$\varkappa, \lambda$	$\varkappa, \lambda$	$\varkappa, \lambda$

Abbreviations: H chain = heavy chain; S value = sedimentation coefficient of a protein as determined by ultracentrifugation; Gm = genetic marker on the γ chain; Am = genetric marker on the α chain; Km = genetic marker on the $\varkappa$ chain; L chain = light chain.

disulfide bridges. Four subclasses of IgG have been identified based on heavy chain differences—γ_1, γ_2, γ_3, and γ_4, which correspond to IgG1, IgG2, IgG3, and IgG4.

2. Biological and chemical properties
   a. IgG has a molecular weight of 150,000 and an S value of 7S.
   b. IgG is the only immunoglobulin that can cross the placenta in humans and, therefore, is responsible for protection of the newborn during the first months of life.
   c. IgG molecules are capable of fixing complement, except for IgG4. The complement binding site is in the C_H2 domain.
   d. As the major antibody in secondary immune responses, IgG has a half-life of approximately 21 days.
   e. IgG is important in phagocytosis (opsonization) since phagocytic cells (e.g., macrophages and neutrophils) have receptors for the Fc fragment of IgG, primarily IgG1 and IgG3.

B. IgA is present in the serum and in various bodily secretions, and thus takes two forms.

   1. Serum IgA accounts for about 15%–20% of the total normal serum immunoglobulin pool and is present at a concentration of approximately 200 mg/dl.
      a. Structure. In humans, over 80% of serum IgA exists in a monomeric form with an S value of 7S, with the rest existing as polymers in the form of dimers, trimers, or tetramers. In polymeric IgA, the monomeric units are linked by disulfide bonds and **joining (J) chain**.
         (1) J chain is a glycopeptide chain with a molecular weight of approximately 15,000 associated with polymeric forms of immunoglobulins that contain two or more basic units (i.e., IgA and IgM).
         (2) It is covalently linked to heavy chains at the carboxy terminal portions of α and μ chains.
      b. Biological and chemical properties
         (1) IgA does not fix complement via the **classical pathway** but may do so via the **alternative pathway** (see Chapter 4, section II). It has a half-life of 5 days.
         (2) Inactivation of IgA can be caused by an IgA protease produced by certain microorganisms (e.g., *Neisseria gonorrhoeae*).

   2. Secretory IgA (sIgA) is the predominant immunoglobulin in various secretions (e.g., saliva; tears; colostrum; and bronchial, genitourinary, and intestinal secretions).
      a. Structurally, sIgA consists of two monomeric units plus J chain and secretory component (Fig. 3-2). It has an S value of 11S.
         (1) Secretory component is a single polypeptide chain, with a molecular weight of 70,000–75,000 associated with sIgA. It serves as a receptor for IgA as IgA is released from submucosal plasma cells (which also secrete J chain) and diffuses toward the epithelial cells.
         (2) The dominant subclass of sIgA is **IgA2**, which is unique for its absence of a covalent bond between the light and heavy chains. In this subclass, light chains are linked by disulfide bonds, which is the form of sIgA shown in Figure 3-2.

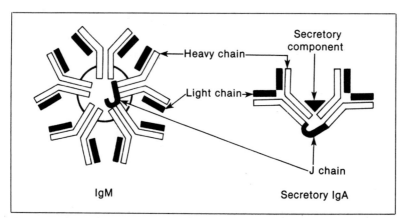

IgM   Secretory IgA

Figure 3-2. Structural models of IgM and secretory IgA. IgM has a pentameric structure linked by J chain at the Fc fragment. Secretory IgA has a dimeric structure plus J chain plus secretory component, and is shown in the dominant IgA2 subclass, which is unique for its absence of a covalent bond between the light and heavy chains. Light chains are linked by disulfide bonds.

b. Biological and chemical properties
   (1) Secretory component is synthesized by epithelial cells and enables IgA to pass through the mucosal tissues into the secretions. It appears to protect IgA from proteolysis.
   (2) IgA has a half-life of approximately 5–6 days; sIgA is responsible for local immunity.
   (3) The sIgA molecules protect mucosal surfaces by reacting with the surface of potential pathogens and interfering with their adherence and colonization.

C. IgM represents about 8%–10% of the total serum immunoglobulins and is present in normal serum at a concentration of approximately 120 mg/dl.

   1. Structure. With an S value of 19S, IgM has a pentameric structure, consisting of five monomeric units linked by J chain and disulfide bonds at the Fc fragment (Fig. 3-2). IgM is easily dissociated by reducing agents, forming five monomeric units of 7S IgM.

   2. Biological and chemical properties
      a. IgM is the predominant antibody in the early (primary) immune response to most antigens and the predominant antibody produced by the fetus. An elevated IgM level in cord serum (normal level, approximately 10 mg/dl) of a newborn may indicate infection in the fetus.
      b. IgM is the most efficient immunoglobulin at fixing complement in lytic reactions and enhancing phagocytosis. It has a half-life of approximately 5 days.
      c. Some IgM is synthesized locally in secretory tissues (e.g., parotid tissue). Secretory IgM, like IgA, has the capacity to bind secretory component.

D. IgD represents less than 1% of the total immunoglobulin pool and is present in trace amounts in normal serum (approximately 3–5 mg/dl).

   1. Structural studies are difficult due to low serum concentrations of IgD and because of its susceptibility to enzymatic degradation. One unique structural feature is the presence of only a single H—H interchain bond, along with two H—L interchain bonds.

   2. Biological and chemical properties
      a. IgD occurs in large quantities on the membrane of human B cells and may, as an antigen receptor, be involved in B-cell activation.
      b. The molecule has been reported to have some antibody activity for penicillin, insulin, and diphtheria toxoid; however, there is still some controversy over its precise biological function.
      c. IgD has a half-life of 2–3 days; it is heat and acid labile.

E. IgE is present in trace amounts in normal serum (approximately 100 ng/ml), accounting for only 0.004% of serum immunoglobulin.

   1. Structure. IgE is a monomer with the unusual feature of the separation of two heavy chain interchain disulfide bonds by one complete domain.

   2. Biological and chemical properties
      a. IgE has a molecular weight of approximately 190,000 and an S value of 8S.
      b. IgE is produced by plasma cells (B cells) in the spleen and lymphoid tissue of the tonsils and adenoids as well as in the respiratory and gastrointestinal mucosa (see also Chapter 9, section II B 2 b). IgE production begins in the fetus very early in the gestational process.
      c. IgE is unique among immunoglobulins in its heat lability (at 56°C). It is unable to fix complement via the classical pathway, and it does not cross the placenta.
      d. IgE is described as **homocytotropic** due to its affinity for cells ("cytotropic") of the host species that produced it ("homo"), particularly for tissue mast cells and blood basophils. Fixation occurs via the Fc fragment (C3 and C4 domains).
      e. Because of its ability to attach to human skin, IgE is associated with immediate hypersensitivity reactions (e.g., atopy and anaphylaxis) but also, apparently, with immunity to certain helminthic parasites. IgE has a vascular half-life of 2–3 days.

IV. ANTIBODY DIVERSITY

A. Allotypic and idiotypic variation. In addition to isotypic (class) variation already described, immunoglobulins also display allotypic and idiotypic variation.

   1. Allotypes are genetic variants of plasma proteins existing in different individuals within the same species that are inherited in a mendelian manner. Allotypic markers are found on heavy and light chains and are localized in the constant region. Nomenclature for allotypic markers have been established for γ, α, and *x* chains. The loci are designated as follows:

a. Markers on γ chains are designated **Gm** (for **g**amma), referring to IgG.

b. Markers on α chains are designated **Am** (for **a**lpha), referring to IgA.

c. Markers on *x* chains are designated **Km**, or **Inv.**

2. **Idiotypes** represent unique antigenic determinants, or amino acid sequences in the variable region, associated with the antigen-binding capability of the molecule. They are usually specific for the individual antibody clone (**private idiotypes**) but may be shared among different clones (**public idiotypes**). **Idiotypic variability** pertains to the generation of the antigen-combining site in the variable region of the heavy and light chains. Variability in amino acid sequence in these regions is concentrated in three to four hypervariable regions ("hot spots") surrounded by relatively invariant residues (see section II C 1). These regions are the areas that make contact with the antigen.

B. **Gene organization.** Immunoglobulin gene organization is studied in order to establish the role of immunoglobulin inheritance. Part of the variability in immunoglobulin structure stems from the interaction of the individual chains.

1. **Separate diversity exists for each chain** since they are coded for on separate **chromosomes.** In the human they are:

a. Heavy chain: chromosome 14

b. Light (λ) chain: chromosome 22

c. Light (*x*) chain: chromosome 2

2. The heavy and light chains vary markedly in amino acid composition of their amino terminal portion (variable region) but are relatively constant in their carboxy terminal portion (constant region). Analysis of immunoglobulin genes has revealed that the variable and constant regions are separately encoded and located on different fragments of DNA.

3. **Light chain gene organization.** Three genes code for each immunoglobulin light chain, as discussed below using the human *x* chain as an example (Fig. 3-3).

a. One gene controls the variable domain. The initial gene segment, the variable (V_x) region, codes for the first 95 amino acids of the variable region protein. Multiple V_x regions exist.

b. A second gene codes for a small peptide that occurs at the junction of the variable and constant regions. These remaining 13 amino acids (96–108) of the variable portion are contributed by one of five segments called **joining** (J_x) segments.

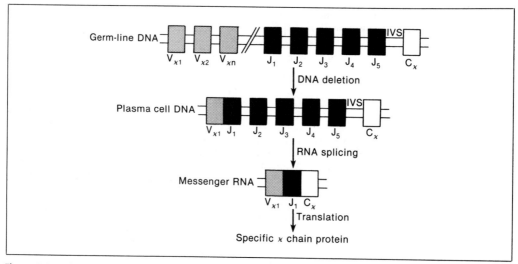

Figure 3-3. Light (*x*) chain gene organization. The potential for a large variety of *x* chains exists due to somatic recombination in the DNA and to RNA splicing. As the germ-line DNA differentiates into a plasma cell, DNA deletion brings one of the variable (V_x) genes next to one of the joining (*J*) genes—in this example, V_{x1} and J_1. This unit and the remaining J genes are separated from the constant (C_x) region by an intervening sequence (*IVS*) of DNA. The V_{x1}–J_1 unit codes for one of the numerous possible *x* chain variable regions. The plasma cell DNA is transcribed into nuclear RNA, which is spliced to form messenger RNA, with V_{x1}, J_1 and C_x joined and ready for translation into *x* chain. (Adapted from David J: Antibodies, structure and function. In *Scientific American: Medicine,* vol 1, sect 6. New York, Scientific American, 1987, p 16.)

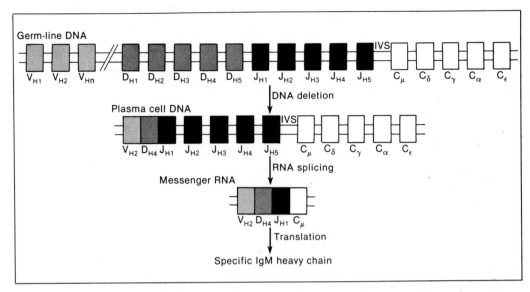

Figure 3-4. Heavy (μ) chain organization. The potential for variety in heavy chains, as in $\varkappa$ chains, is due to somatic recombination in the DNA and to RNA splicing. As the germ-line DNA differentiates into a plasma cell, DNA deletion brings one of the variable (V_H) genes, one of the diversity (D_H) genes, and one of the joining (J_H) genes together—in this example, V_{H2}, D_{H4}, and J_{H1}. This unit and the remaining J genes are separated from the constant (C) region by an intervening sequence (*IVS*). The plasma cell DNA is transcribed into nuclear RNA, which is spliced to form messenger RNA. In this process, the C_μ gene is selected and joined to the V_{H2}–D_{H4}–J_{H1} complex, and the entire unit is ready for translation into μ chain. (Adapted from David J: Antibodies, structure and function. In *Scientific American:Medicine*, vol 1, sect 6. New York, 1987, p 17.)

      c. A third gene dictates the amino acid sequence of the constant region. There is only one constant $\varkappa$ ($C_\varkappa$) region on this final segment, which codes for amino acids 109–214.

  4. Heavy chain gene organization is discussed below using the heavy chain of IgM (Fig. 3-4).
      a. Although similar to that of light chain genes, heavy chain gene organization is more complex in that **three**, not two, **segments of DNA**, join to generate a gene coding for the variable portion of the heavy chain: V_H, D_H, and J_H. The additional germ-line gene segment is designated the **diversity (D_H) gene region**.
      b. The D_H segment accounts for the third hypervariable region of the heavy chain. The D segment, in conjunction with the variable and joining segments, is utilized to generate the enormous diversity of the heavy chain.

C. Genetic mechanisms contribute to the generation of the total pool of antibody specificities of a given host.

  1. Germ-line theory. A large amount of antibody diversity is created by chance recombination, as illustrated in Figures 3-3 and 3-4 by the DNA–RNA mechanism. As a result of somatic recombination in the DNA and of RNA splicing, more than 1500 varieties of light chains and more than 5000 varieties of heavy chains can be produced.

  2. Somatic mutation theory. Further diversity could result from extensive point mutations involving a small number of germ-line genes (the **somatic mutation theory**). The theory suggests that a small number of germ-line genes diversify either by point mutations or by recombination events during lymphocyte differentiation. Present evidence suggests strongly that both germ-line genes and somatically mutated genes contribute to antibody diversity.

STUDY QUESTIONS

Directions: The question below contains five suggested answers. Choose the **one best** response to the question.

1. In comparison to the other classes of immunoglobulins, IgM is predominant in all of the following ways EXCEPT

(A) complement fixation
(B) primary immune response to most antigens
(C) enhancing phagocytosis
(D) production by the fetus
(E) heat sensitivity

Directions: Each question below contains four suggested answers of which **one or more** is correct. Choose the answer

A   if **1, 2, and 3** are correct
B   if **1 and 3** are correct
C   if **2 and 4** are correct
D   if **4** is correct
E   if **1, 2, 3, and 4** are correct

2. Components of an Fab fragment include

(1) an entire light chain
(2) the V_H and C_H1 domains of the heavy chain
(3) the Fd fragment
(4) the carboxy terminal portion of the heavy chain

3. Idiotypic variability pertains to the generation of the antigen-combining site in the

(1) constant region of the heavy chain
(2) variable region of the heavy chain
(3) C_H1 domain of the heavy chain
(4) variable region of the light chain

4. The variable portion of the IgM heavy chain is generated by segments of DNA including

(1) V_H
(2) J_H
(3) D_H
(4) C_μ

5. J chain is a glycopeptide chain associated with which of the following immunoglobulins?

(1) IgA
(2) IgG
(3) IgM
(4) IgE

6. Basic structural units of an immunoglobulin molecule include

(1) identical x or λ light chains
(2) one constant and three variable regions
(3) two identical heavy and two identical light chains
(4) a total of five domains

7. Characteristics of IgE, the immunoglobulin involved in atopy allergy, include

(1) J chain as part of the molecule
(2) ability to cross the placenta
(3) ability to activate complement via the classical pathway
(4) affinity for cells of the host

Directions: The groups of questions below consist of lettered choices followed by several numbered items. For each numbered item select the **one** lettered choice with which it is **most** closely associated. Each lettered choice may be used once, more than once, or not at all.

Questions 8–13

For each characteristic, select the immuno-globulin it most appropriately describes.

(A) IgE
(B) IgA
(C) IgG
(D) IgM
(E) IgD

C 8. Half-life of approximately 21 days.

D 9. Elevated level in cord serum of a newborn, which may indicate infection

A 10. Immediate hypersensitivity

B 11. Predominant immunoglobulin in various secretions

D 12. Predominant antibody in the early (primary) immune response

C 13. Crosses the placenta in humans

Questions 14–18

Match the descriptions with the labeled areas in the diagram.

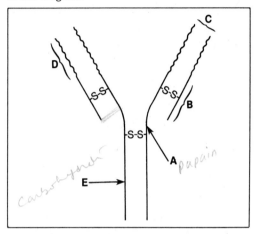

A 14. Site where papain cleaves the IgG molecule

E 15. Point of attachment of carbohydrate on heavy chain

C 16. Area of Ig molecule where antigen attaches

B 17. Constant region of light chain

D 18. Variable region of light chain

ANSWERS AND EXPLANATIONS

1. The answer is E. (*III C*) IgM is a cyclic pentamer consisting of five basic units linked by joining (J) chain at the Fc fragment. Because of its relatively high valence (theoretically 10), it is the most efficient immunoglobulin at fixing complement and enhancing phagocytosis. IgM antibodies form a major proportion of the primary immune response, whereas the secondary response consists almost entirely of IgG. IgM is synthesized before birth and represents the predominant antibody produced by the fetus. It is not heat sensitive as is IgE.

2. The answer is A (1, 2, 3). (*II E 1 a, b*) Treatment of the monomeric basic unit with the enzyme papain splits it into two Fab (antigen-binding) and one Fc (crystallizable) fragments. Each monovalent Fab fragment contains an entire light chain and the V_H and C_H1 domains of the heavy chain, referred to as the Fd fragment. The Fc fragment contains the carboxy terminal portion of the heavy chain.

3. The answer is C (2, 4). (*IV A 2*) Idiotypes represent unique amino acid sequences involved in the generation of the antigen-combining site in the variable region of the heavy and light chains. Variability in amino acid sequence in these regions is concentrated in hypervariable regions ("hot spots"). The constant region of the heavy chain, including the C_H1 domain, demonstrates an unvarying amino acid sequence except for isotypic and allotypic variations.

4. The answer is A (1, 2, 3). (*IV B 4*) In IgM heavy chain gene organization, three (V_H, D_H, J_H) segments of DNA join together to generate the variable portion of the heavy chain. The D_H segment accounts for the third hypervariable region of the heavy chain. The C_μ segment of DNA codes for the constant region of heavy chain.

5. The answer is B (1, 3). [*III B 1 b (1), (2), C 1*] Joining (J) chain is a glycopeptide chain associated with polymeric forms of immunoglobulins that contain two or more basic units (e.g., IgA and IgM). It is linked to heavy chains at the carboxy terminal portion of α and μ chains. IgG and IgE exist as monomeric forms and hence contain no J chain.

6. The answer is B (1, 3). (*II B 2*) The basic structural unit (monomer) of immunoglobulin molecules consists of four polypeptide chains, two identical heavy and two identical light chains. Light chains are of either the x or λ type. A given molecule always contains identical x or λ chains, never a mixture of the two. Each of the four chains has a variable (amino terminal) portion and a constant (carboxy terminal) portion plus either two (light chains), four (γ, α, and δ heavy chains), or five (μ and ϵ heavy chains) domains.

7. The answer is D (4). (*III E 1, 2 a–e*) The basic structural unit of immunoglobulin molecules is called a monomer. Human immunoglobulins may appear as monomers, dimers, or pentamers; the polymeric immunoglobulins are formed with glycopeptide chains called J chains. IgE is a monomer and, therefore, does not contain a J chain as part of the molecule. Unlike IgG, IgE does not cross the placenta; however, IgE production begins in the fetus very early in the gestational process. IgE is described as homocytotropic due to its affinity for cells of the host species that produced it; because of its ability to attach to human skin, IgE is associated with immediate hypersensitivity reactions (anaphylaxis, atopic allergy). IgE is unable to fix complement via the classical pathway.

8–13. The answers are: 8-C, 9-D, 10-A, 11-B, 12-D, 13-C. (*III A–E*) IgE is associated with immediate types of hypersensitivity reactions (e.g., atopy and anaphylaxis) but also, apparently, with immunity to certain helminthic parasites. IgA is the predominant immunoglobulin in various secretions (e.g., saliva, tears, and colostrum), is referred to as secretory IgA (sIgA), and consists of two basic units plus joining (J) chain and secretory component. IgG, the major immunoglobulin in normal human serum (approximately 75% of the total), has a half-life of approximately 21 days, the longest of any of the immunoglobulins. It is the only immunoglobulin that can cross the placenta in humans, thus protecting the newborn during the first months of life. IgM is the predominant antibody in the early (primary) immune response and the predominant antibody produced by the fetus. An elevated IgM level in cord serum (normal level, 10 mg/dl) of a newborn may indicate an infection in the fetus.

14–18. The answers are: 14-A, 15-E, 16-C, 17-B, 18-D. (*II C 1–2; E 1 b, 2; Fig. 3-1*) Papain cleaves the IgG molecule into three fragments of approximately equal size at the hinge region. The Fc fragment, or carboxy terminal portion of the heavy chain, contains carbohydrate. The Fab fragments, each containing an entire light chain and the V_H and C_H1 domains of heavy chain, bind antigen. The variable region of light chains is at the amino, or N, terminal portion of the molecule; the constant region is at the carboxy, or C, terminal portion.

4

The Complement System

I. THE COMPLEMENT SYSTEM plays a major role in host defense and the inflammatory process. Complement consists of a complex series of at least 15 plasma proteins that normally are functionally inactive.

  A. Major functions. Activation of the complement system results in the generation of a wide range of biological activities that can be divided into three major functions.

   1. Opsonic function. Following activation, opsonization occurs as complement components coat pathogenic organisms or immune complexes, facilitating the process of phagocytosis.

   2. Inflammatory function. Activation of the complement system results in induction of histamine release from mast cells and basophils and stimulation of the inflammatory response.

   3. Cytotoxic function. In the final stage of the complement cascade, membrane attack of target cells (e.g., bacteria and tumor cells) occurs, leading to cell death.

  B. Complement component nomenclature. The complement system is made up of nine major complement components (Table 4-1) designated by **C** followed by an identifying numeral from 1 to 9 (e.g., C1, C2). The numerals indicate the order in which components are activated.*

   1. Peptide chains of each component are designated by Greek letters (e.g., C3α, C4β).

   2. Cleaved peptides from fragmented peptide chains are denoted by lowercase letters (e.g., C3a).

   3. If further proteolysis results in loss of fragment activity, a subscript **i** is added to indicate inactivation (e.g., C3b$_i$).

   4. When a complement protein acquires enzymatic activity, a horizontal bar is indicated over the numeral of the component (e.g., C$\overline{1}$) or over numerals of component complexes (e.g., C$\overline{5b67}$) in the case of a nonenzymatic activated state.

II. PATHWAYS OF ACTIVATION. Complement is activated sequentially in a cascading manner, with a protein being activated only by the protein that directly preceded it in the sequence. Activation may occur via two pathways, the **classical** and the **alternative pathways**. The classical pathway involves a more recently evolved mechanism of specific adaptive immunity, whereas the alternative pathway provides nonspecific innate immunity.

  A. The classical pathway requires the interaction of all nine major complement components.

   1. Activation of the classical pathway may occur via **antigen–antibody complexes** or by aggregated **immunoglobulins**.
      a. IgG (mainly IgG$_1$, IgG$_2$, and IgG$_3$) and IgM are most efficient in reacting with complement. Only one molecule of IgM is required, whereas at least two molecules of IgG are needed. Activation follows binding of complement to a site (C$_H$2 domain on IgG; C$_H$4 on IgM) on the Fc fragment of the immunoglobulin.
      b. Classically, an antigen–antibody complex is designated by **EA**, where E is the antigen (erythrocyte in the original historical observations) and A is the antibody.
         (1) Other antigens can substitute for E; thus, EA might represent immune complexes or antibody-coated bacteria, tumor cells, or lymphocytes.

---

*Component C4 is activated out of numerical order; components were assigned numbers in the order in which they were discovered, not in sequential order.

Table 4-1. Properties of Complement Components

Component	Serum Concentration (μg/ml)	Activation Products	Molecular Weight
Classical pathway			
C1q	180		410,000
C1r	50		170,000
		C1̄r	170,000
C1s	100		85,000
		C1̄s	85,000
C4	500		210,000
		C4a	10,000
		C4b	200,000
C2	30		115,000
		C2a	80,000
		C2b	35,000
C3	1300		195,000
		C3a	9000
		C3b	186,000
Alternative pathway			
B	200		93,000
		Ba	30,000
		Bb	63,000
D	1–5		25,000
		D̄	25,000
P	25		184,000
Common pathway			
C5	75		205,000
		C5a	11,000
		C5b	195,000
C6	60		128,000
C7	55		121,000
C8	80		155,000
C9	200		75,000
Regulatory proteins			
C1̄ INH	180		100,000
C3b INA	25		100,000
C4b-binding protein	?		540,000
β1H	670		150,000

After Porter RR, Reid KBM: Activation of the complement system by antibody–antigen complexes: the classical pathway. *Adv Prot Chem* 33:1–71, 1979.

(2) Complement components bind to EA in an orderly sequence to form a macromolecular complex, **EAC 142356789**. The numerals indicate the order in which components bind to the complex.

2. Components. The classical pathway involves the following components and steps (Fig. 4-1).
 a. C1. When IgG or IgM reacts with antigen, the Fc fragment of the immunoglobulin provides a C1 binding site. C1, also called the **recognition unit**, contains three polypeptides—C1q, C1r, and C1s—that are held together by **calcium ions**. With the removal of the calcium, C1 breaks down into its three subunits.
  (1) C1q, the portion of the molecule that attaches first to immunoglobulin and initiates complement activation, has six binding sites. Because of its multivalency it can cross-link multiple immunoglobulin molecules.
  (2) C1q binding leads to activation of C1r proenzymes.

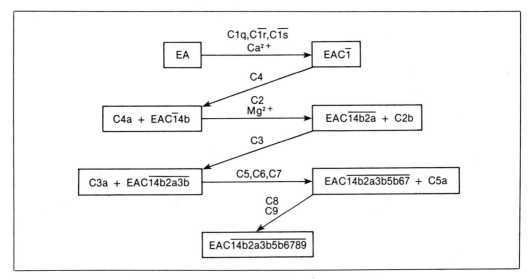

Figure 4-1. Classical pathway of complement activation.

(3) Activated **C$\overline{1}$r** cleaves the proenzyme **C1s**. The latter acquires esterase activity and is referred to as **C$\overline{1}$ esterase (C$\overline{1}$s)**.Calcium ions are essential for activation of C1.

b. C4. C$\overline{1}$s mediates cleavage of native C4, the next component in the complement cascade, into C4a and C4b. One molecule of C$\overline{1}$s can cleave several C4 molecules, thus serving as one of the sites in the amplification process.

  (1) C4a, one of three **anaphylatoxins**, is released into the fluid phase.

  (2) C4b can bind to cell membranes. The binding of C4b to membranes is rather inefficient, but several C4b molecules may cluster about C$\overline{1}$s on the membrane surface.

c. C2. C$\overline{1}$s in the presence of C4b cleaves the next component, C2, into C2a and C2b.

  (1) C2a remains linked to the cell-bound C4b, thus forming the bimolecular complex **C4b2a**. **Magnesium ions** are required for formation of the C$\overline{4b2a}$ complex. C$\overline{4b2a}$ has enzymatic activity and is referred to as classical pathway **C3 convertase**.

  (2) C2b is released into the fluid phase.

d. C3. The substrate for C3 convertase is C3. Circulating C3 binds to the C$\overline{4b2a}$ complex and is cleaved into two fragments, C3a and C3b.

  (1) C3a is an anaphylatoxin and remains unbound.

  (2) C3b is bound to the membrane in the vicinity of the C$\overline{4b2a}$ complex (C3 convertase), forming a trimolecular complex, **C4b2a3b**, which has enzymatic activity. The C$\overline{4b2a3b}$ complex is also referred to as **C5 convertase**, which acts on C5, the first complement component of the **membrane attack pathway**.

B. The alternative pathway, also referred to as the **properdin pathway**, is considered to be a primitive defense system, a bypass mechanism that does not require C1, C4, and C2 interaction.

 1. Activation can be triggered **immunologically** (e.g., by IgA and some IgG) and **nonimmunologically** [e.g., by certain microbial cell surfaces, complex polysaccharides, and bacterial lipopolysaccharides (endotoxin)].

 2. Components. The alternative pathway involves the following components and steps (Fig. 4-2).

  a. C3. The initial recognition event necessary for alternative pathway activation is the presence of C3, specifically **C3b**, which is probably continuously generated in small amounts in the circulation.

   (1) If C3b binds to a **nonactivator** (nonprotected) surface, it binds to **factor H (β1H)** and becomes inactivated through combined actions of factor H and **factor I [C3b inactivator (C3b INA)]**.

   (2) If C3b binds to an **activator** (protected) surface, its ability to bind to factor H is diminished.

  b. Factor B. The surface-bound, protected C3b interacts with factor B, also called the **C3 proactivator**, to form **C3b,B**, which is a magnesium ion-dependent complex.

  c. Factor $\overline{D}$. The complex C3b,B is susceptible to enzymatic cleavage by factor $\overline{D}$, also called **C3 proactivator convertase**, into two fragments, Ba and Bb.

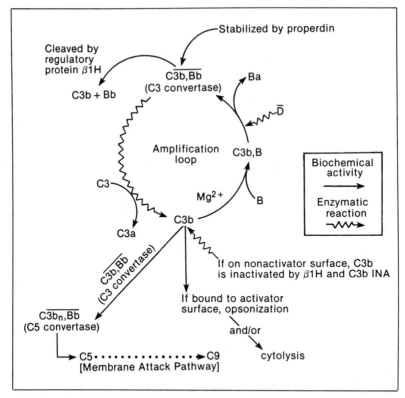

Figure 4-2. Alternative pathway of complement activation.

   (1) The **Ba** fragment is released.
   (2) An active site is exposed in the **Bb** fragment, which remains bound to C3b, forming the **C3b,Bb** complex, also called **amplification C3 convertase.** When stabilized by the binding of **properdin (P)**, which slows the dissociation of Bb, the C3b,Bb complex becomes a **C3 convertase** that cleaves C3 and generates more C3b. C3b then fixes to the activator surface so that more factor B binding sites are exposed, and the amplification loop amplifies the initial recognition event.
   d. As more C3b is generated, the complex expands (**$\overline{\text{C3b}_n,\text{Bb}}$**; where $n > 1$) and becomes a **C5 convertase** capable of cleaving C5 into C5a and C5b and initiating the membrane attack pathway.
   e. Cobra venom factor (CVF) contained in cobra venom has the interesting property of activating the alternative complement pathway. Like C3b, it complexes with Bb to form CVF,Bb which is resistant to factors H and I and capable of continuously activating the C3-to-C3b conversion leading to complement depletion.

III. THE PATHWAY OF MEMBRANE ATTACK, also called the **common pathway**, is marked by the convergence of the classical and alternative pathways at the point of C5 activation.

   A. Activation of the **membrane attack complex** is initiated by C5 convertase (i.e., $\overline{\text{C4b2a3b}}$ in the classical pathway and $\overline{\text{C3b}_n,\text{Bb}}$ in the alternative pathway). This is the only component in the attack complex that has enzymatic activity, with cleavage occurring only once. All other components bind spontaneously.

   B. Components. The membrane attack complex involves the following components and steps.

   1. C5 is cleaved by C5 convertase into a smaller C5a fragment and a larger C5b fragment.
       a. C5a, an anaphylatoxin, is released into the surrounding fluid medium.
       b. C5b is the first component of the membrane attack complex. It is the receptor for the C6 and C7 components.

   2. C6 and C7. Unstable C5b binds to C6, forming a stable C5b6 complex, which subsequently binds to C7, forming the metastable trimolecular **$\overline{\text{C5b67}}$** complex that is bound to the target cell membrane.

3. **C8** attaches to the membrane-bound C5b67 complex and membrane leakage begins. **Cell lysis** can occur by the C5b678 complex in the absence of C9.

4. **C9** attachment to the C5b678 complex serves a primary function of greatly **accelerating cytolysis** by the production of circular lesions in the membrane.

C. **Cell lysis.** The C5b6789 complex induces the formation of **hollow cylinders** (tubules) about 15 nm long and 8–12 nm in diameter in the lipid bilayer of the cell membrane, allowing passage of electrolytes and water across the membrane and leading ultimately to osmotic lysis of the cell.

IV. **REGULATORY MECHANISMS.** Activation of the complement components is associated with potent biological functions that, if left unchecked, would exhaust the complement system. Uncontrolled activation of the complement system is prevented by several serum proteins that bind to (inhibit) or enzymatically attack (inactivate) complement components.

A. **Inhibitor**

1. **C1 esterase inhibitor (C1 INH)** is a plasma α_2-globulin that inhibits the enzymatic activity of C1 esterase by dissociating the subunits C1q, C1r, and C1s.
   a. It also inhibits plasmin, kallikrein, activated Hageman factor, and factor XI.
   b. Deficiency of C1 INH results in hereditary angioedema, an inherited defect characterized by transient but recurrent episodes of local edema.

B. **Inactivators**

1. **Factor I** (C3b INA) is a serum enzyme that cleaves C3b free in solution or on the surface of cells. The degradation products are unable to function in the C4b2a3b complex. One degradation product, **C3c**, is converted to **C3e**.

2. **Factor H** ($\beta 1H$) acts in concert with factor I to cleave the alpha chain of C3b, leading to formation of cleavage product **C3b$_i$**, which no longer interacts with the alternative pathway components.

3. **Anaphylatoxin inactivator** is an α-globulin that enzymatically destroys the biological activity of C3a, C4a, and C5a by removing the molecules' carboxyl terminal arginine.

4. **C4 binding protein (C4Bp)** is a serum protein that controls the activity of cell-bound C4b. Like the interaction of factor H and C3b, it binds to C4b and allows cleavage (alpha chain) and destruction of C4b by C3b INA.

V. **BIOLOGICAL CONSEQUENCES OF COMPLEMENT ACTIVATION.** During complement activation, a number of materials with important biological activities are generated.

A. **C3 and C5** and their cleavage products appear to be the most important complement components in terms of biological function.

1. **C3a and C5a** are referred to as anaphylatoxins.
   a. They cause the **release of vasoactive amines** (e.g., histamine) from mast cells and basophils in a manner that simulates mediator release by IgE.
   b. Mediator release causes **smooth muscle contraction** and **increases vascular permeability**, effects which can be counteracted by antihistamines and anaphylatoxin inactivator. C3a and C5a also appear to have the ability to contract smooth muscle and increase capillary permeability **directly** (i.e., without the mediation of mast cells and basophils).
   c. C3a appears to function as an **immunoregulatory molecule**, demonstrating immunosuppressive activity in both antigen-specific and mitogen-induced immunoglobulin synthesis.
   d. C5a is much more active than C3a on a molar basis and, in addition to anaphylatoxin activity, has a wider range of biological activity, including the following.
      (1) It seems to be the major complement-derived **chemotactic factor** in serum, causing the directed migration of neutrophils toward the site where it is generated.
      (2) It causes neutrophils to adhere to the endothelium of vessels and to one another, leading to **neutropenia**.
      (3) It activates neutrophils, triggering a bactericidal **oxidative burst** and **degranulation**.
      (4) It stimulates production of **leukotrienes** [e.g., slow-reacting substance of anaphylaxis (SRS-A)] by neutrophils.
      (5) It loses anaphylatoxin activity but retains chemotactic and neutrophil activating ability after removal of carboxyl terminal arginine (C5a-des-arg) by anaphylatoxin inactivator.

2. **C3b generation and coating** on target cells is perhaps the major biological function of complement.

    a. Its role in the **activation of the alternative complement pathway** has been described (see section II B 2 a).

    b. C3b also plays an important role in **opsonization**.

      (1) Several cell types have surface receptors for C3b, including neutrophils, eosinophils, monocytes and macrophages, B cells, basophils, and primate erythrocytes.

      (2) In the case of phagocytic cells, contact of C3b-coated particles (e.g., bacteria, antigen–antibody complexes) with the cell surface promotes attachment and ultimate ingestion of the particles.

      (3) C3b-coated cells also tend to aggregate (**immune adherence**), a process that also may promote phagocytosis.

    c. The biological significance of the presence of C3b receptors on B cells is not entirely clear, but they may play a role in the induction of certain humoral immune responses.

  3. **C3e** is derived by proteolytic cleavage from C3c which, in turn, is derived from C3b by the action of factor H and factor I. C3e provokes a release of neutrophils from bone marrow, causing prompt **leukocytosis**.

  4. **C3d**, another cleavage product of C3b, can interact with receptors on lymphocytes.

  5. **C3 nephritic factor (C3NeF)** is a pathologic component of the alternative pathway found in the circulation of patients with **mesangiocapillary glomerulonephritis**. It acts as an antibody against the $\overline{C3b,Bb}$ complex and leads to a marked **hypocomplementemia**.

  6. **The $\overline{C5b67}$ complex** has also been reported to have **chemotactic activity**. In serum, however, it is rapidly inactivated and hence it is not yet clear whether the complex plays an important chemotactic role.

B. **C4** and its cleavage products have certain important biological functions.

  1. Activated C4 molecules attach to membranes in close proximity to the C1 site. The binding of C1 and C4 by a virus–antibody complex can **neutralize virus activity**. It is probable that the C4 molecules prevent viral attachment to target cells.

  2. **C4a**, a cleavage fragment of C4 released during activation, has been shown to have **anaphylatoxin activity**, causing the release of histamine from mast cells and basophils.

  3. **C4b receptor sites** exist on several cell types (e.g., phagocytic cells, lymphocytes, and primate erythrocytes), suggesting a role for C4b in **opsonization** as seen with C3b.

C. **C2** cleavage has been reported to be linked to the production of a kinin-like molecule that increases vascular permeability and contracts smooth muscle. It is thought to be involved in the symptoms seen in **hereditary angioedema**, a disease caused by uncontrolled $\overline{C1s}$ activity due to deficiency in $\overline{C1}$ INH.

D. **Ba and Bb.** Two factors generated exclusively by the alternative pathway have important biological functions.

  1. Ba is chemotactic for neutrophils.

  2. Bb activates macrophages and causes them to adhere to and spread on surfaces.

E. **Immunodeficiencies** result from a lack of complement and faulty complement activation (see Chapter 11).

STUDY QUESTIONS

Directions: Each question below contains four suggested answers of which **one or more** is correct. Choose the answer

A   if **1, 2, and 3** are correct
B   if **1 and 3** are correct
C   if **2 and 4** are correct
D   if **4** is correct
E   if **1, 2, 3, and 4** are correct

1.   Complement components not required in the alternative pathway include

(1) C4
(2) C2
(3) C1
(4) C3

2.   Anaphylatoxin inactivator is a serum enzyme that destroys the biological activity of

(1) C2a
(2) C5a
(3) C1a
(4) C3a

3.   C5a stimulates neutrophils to

(1) migrate
(2) adhere to the endothelium of vessels
(3) trigger an oxidative burst
(4) produce leukotrienes

4.   Factor I is a serum enzyme that

(1) enhances opsonization
(2) destroys anaphylatoxin inactivator
(3) enhances immune adherence
(4) cleaves C3b

5.   True statements concerning C3 nephritic factor include which of the following?

(1) It is a pathologic component of the alternative complement pathway
(2) It is important in neutralizing virus activity
(3) It is antibody against the C3b,Bb complex
(4) It is essential for release of neutrophils from bone marrow

6.   Magnesium ions are required for the formation of

(1) the factor H binding site
(2) C1 esterase
(3) factor A
(4) the C4b2a complex

Directions: The group of questions below consists of lettered choices followed by several numbered items. For each numbered item select the **one** lettered choice with which it is **most** closely associated. Each lettered choice may be used once, more than once, or not at all.

Questions 7–11

For each complement component characteristic, select the component that is associated with it.

(A) C2
(B) C4
(C) C3b,Bb
(D) C3e
(E) C3b

7. Neutralizes virus activities

8. Stabilized by properdin

9. Causes symptoms seen in hereditary angioedema

10. Provokes release of neutrophils from bone marrow

11. Promotes opsonization

ANSWERS AND EXPLANATIONS

1. The answer is A (1, 2, 3). (*II B*) The alternative pathway of complement activation, also referred to as the properdin pathway, is considered to be a primitive defense system, a bypass mechanism that does not require C1, C4, and C2 interaction. The initial requirement is the presence of C3, specifically C3b.

2. The answer is C (2, 4). [*II A 2 b (1), d (1); III B 1 a; IV B 3*] C3a and C5a, as well as C4a, are referred to as anaphylatoxins. They cause release of vasoactive amines from mast cells and basophils, which, in turn, cause smooth muscle contraction and increased vascular permeability. Anaphylatoxin inactivator removes the carboxyl terminal arginine residue from the fragments, destroying their biological activity.

3. The answer is E (all). [*V A 1 d (1)–(4)*] In addition to anaphylatoxin activity, C5a seems to be the major complement-derived chemotactic factor in serum, causing directed migration of neutrophils. It also causes neutrophils to adhere to the endothelial lining of vessels, activates neutrophils towards an oxidative burst, and stimulates neutrophils to produce leukotrienes (e.g., SRS-A).

4. The answer is D (4). (*IV B 1*) Factor I, also known as C3b inactivator (C3b INA), is a serum enzyme that cleaves C3b free in solution or on the surface of cells, rendering it unable to function in either the classical or alternative complement pathway. Opsonization and immune adherence, therefore, are inhibited.

5. The answer is B (1, 3). (*V A 5*) C3 nephritic factor (C3NeF) is a pathologic component of the alternative complement pathway found in the circulation of patients with mesangiocapillary glomerulonephritis. It is an antibody against the $\overline{C3b,Bb}$ complex and leads to a marked hypocomplementemia.

6. The answer is D (4). [*II A 2 c (1)*] In the classical complement pathway, magnesium ions are required for formation of the $\overline{C4b2a}$ complex, the classical pathway C3 convertase. In the alternative pathway, surface-bound, protected C3b interacts with factor B to form $C3b,B$ which is also a magnesium ion-dependent complex. Calcium ions are essential for activation of $C\overline{1}$ esterase in the classical pathway.

7–11. The answers are: 7-B, 8-C, 9-A, 10-D, 11-E. [*V B 1, II B 2 c (2), V C, A 3, A 2 b*] C2 cleavage has been reported to be linked to the production of a kinin-like molecule that increases vascular permeability and contracts smooth muscle. It is thought to be involved in hereditary angioedema, a disease caused by uncontrolled $C\overline{1}s$ activity.

The binding of C1 and C4 by a virus–antibody complex can neutralize virus activity. It is probable that the C4 prevents viral attachment to target cells.

In the alternative pathway, the C3b,B complex is cleaved by factor $\overline{D}$. The Ba fragment is released and the $\overline{C3b,Bb}$ complex, stabilized by properdin, becomes a C3 convertase.

C3e is derived, by proteolytic cleavage, from C3c, which, in turn, is derived from C3b. It provokes a release of neutrophils from the bone marrow, causing prompt leukocytosis.

C3b plays an important role in opsonization.

5
The Immune
Response System

I. INTRODUCTION. When an individual is exposed to antigenic materials, either by injection or infection, a complex series of events ensue, the end result of which will be the production of specific antibodies and antigen-reactive lymphocytes.

    A. The lymphoid cells of the immune system will acquire the ability to recognize a particular antigen. The panorama unfolds when one considers the end result of the interaction of the lymphocyte with its homologous epitopes.

        1. Some cells will be induced to proliferate and differentiate into **plasma cells**. Consider, for example, the possible production of all five classes of immunoglobulins (Ig) [see Chapter 3, section III]. When this potential is multiplied by the number of known subclasses, the possibility emerges for the production of ten distinct proteins (antibodies) in response to a single epitope.

        2. The **lymphocytic responses** to antigen exposure are similarly diverse. Thymic lymphocytes will be induced to differentiate and proliferate to form mature progeny that will be triggered to release biologically active metabolites into the environment when they contact antigen a second time.

    B. The immune response is under extremely complex **genetic control** (see Chapter 3, section IV; Chapter 12, section II B 3).

        1. Three genes code for each immunoglobulin light chain (V, J, and C). Four genes code for each heavy chain (V, J, D, and C).

        2. Further, antibody reactivity is extremely specific, which necessitates that most of these genes must be **polycistronic** (i.e., present in the cell in multiple forms).

        3. The ability to respond to antigens is also under genetic control. The genes that control responsiveness are in the **major histocompatibility complex (MHC)** [see Chapter 12], found in humans on the sixth chromosome, at a locus referred to as Ir (for immune response).

II. COMMON CHARACTERISTICS OF THE LYMPHOID SYSTEM

    A. The lymphoid system involves organs and tissues where lymphocytic cells originate as lymphocyte precursors, then mature and differentiate, and finally lodge in the lymphoid organs or move throughout the body.

        1. Precursor cells originate in the yolk sac, liver, spleen, or bursa of Fabricius (or its mammalian equivalent, the bone marrow) in an embryo or fetus.

        2. Stem cells from bone marrow or embryonic tissues are deposited and mature into lymphocytes in the **central** or **primary lymphoid organs**, which include the thymus and the bursa or bone marrow.

        3. Upon maturation, the lymphocytes then seed **peripheral** or **secondary lymphoid tissue** (i.e., the lymph nodes, spleen, diffuse lymphoid tissues, and lymphoid follicles) where they undergo further maturation toward immunocompetence and production of humoral antibodies or specifically sensitized lymphocytes.

    B. Two facets of the immune response system

        1. Thymus-dependent system. If the thymus of experimental animals (particularly if they are young) is removed, the immune response (primarily cell-mediated immunity) is depressed. A thymus graft from another animal restores immunocompetence and cellular immunity. Even if the thymus graft is placed in a bag impervious to cells but not to fluids, the response is restored. Epithelial cells of the thymus produce soluble molecules that are involved in immunity. Indeed, there are **thymic hormones** (e.g., **thymopoietin**). The cells produced by the **thymus-dependent system** are called **T lymphocytes (T cells)**.

    2. Thymus-independent system. Discovery of the humoral branch of the immune system came about by an accidental observation in chickens.

        a. A lymphoid organ in chickens known as the bursa of Fabricius has a role in immunity involving humoral immunity or circulating antibodies (e.g., IgG, IgA). Removal of the bursa depresses humoral immunity, but not cellular immunity. This system then is referred to as the **thymus-independent system** or **B-cell system**, and the cells that arise through this pathway are called **B lymphocytes (B cells)**.

        b. Humans have a bursa equivalent that is involved with humoral immunity, but there is argument about its location. There is evidence to indicate it is **gut-associated lymphoid tissue (GALT)**—perhaps Peyer's patches of the intestine, tonsils, and appendix. The fetal liver or bone marrow may also be involved.

C. Compartmentalization. An examination of lymph nodes reveals an anatomic division between the two types of lymphocytes.

    1. The B-cell–dependent regions of the lymph nodes are called **germinal centers** and are the sites of antibody production. They undergo change and enlarge when antigens are introduced. If the bursa is removed, a degradation of this area occurs.

    2. Removal of the thymus causes a degeneration of the thymus-dependent, or **juxtamedullary**, region.

    3. In the spleen, the B cells are located in the white pulp, whereas the T cells ensheath the trabecular arteries prior to these vessels entering the white pulp.

D. Collaboration. When antigen enters a lymph node (or the spleen), it is phagocytized by a **macrophage**. The processed antigen is presented to the lymphocytes on the macrophage membrane.

    1. Antigen-specific **helper T (Th) cells** recognize the antigen, as do plasma cell precursor lymphocytes (B cells).

    2. The three cells interact, perhaps in a tricellular complex, and the B cell undergoes blastogenesis and differentiation.

    3. The interaction of the T cell and the B cell is called **collaboration** (see Fig. 5-1). The end result is a humoral immune response (i.e., antibody synthesis and secretion by plasma cells). Cell-mediated immunity is produced in a similar manner; however, the lymphocytic cells entering into this process are distinct from those collaborating to yield mature plasma cells.

III. BIOLOGY OF THE IMMUNE RESPONSE

A. Fate of antigen

    1. When an antigen is injected **subcutaneously** or **intracutaneously** into an animal, it is carried through the lymphatics to the circulatory system. The first deposition of antigen is in the regional lymph node. This is followed by hyperplasia of the node; it increases in size due to cellular proliferation.

    2. If the antigen is administered **intravenously** or **intraperitoneally**, it locates primarily in the spleen. The same chain of events happens as noted above; the spleen enlarges and becomes hyperplastic due to infiltration and proliferation of cells.

    3. Regardless of the route of injection, the macrophage plays a pivotal role in the preparation of the antigen for presentation to the lymphoid cells.

        a. Cellular antigens are phagocytized and partially digested into smaller, more readily handled fragments.

        b. Antigens in colloidal suspension (e.g., serum proteins) are similarly phagocytized; however, it seems that the undigested portion of these antigens is, in some way, processed intracellularly and reappears on the macrophage membrane to subsequently trigger proliferation and differentiation of specifically reactive lymphocytes.

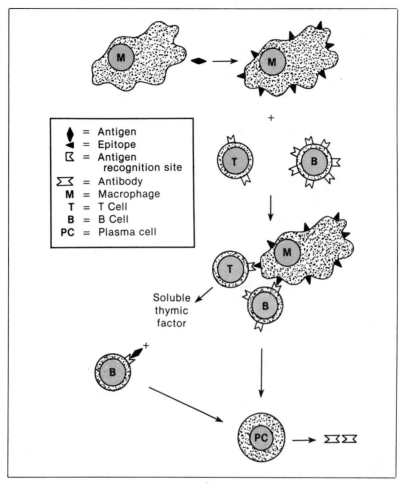

Figure 5-1. Cellular interactions in the humoral immune response. Some antigens do not require participation of T cells.

B. Antibody synthesis

1. Antibody production occurs in **lymphatic tissue**, either in specialized organs such as the spleen or at sites of inflammation.

2. **Plasma cells** are responsible for antibody synthesis; small (6–8 μ) lymphocytes are the precursors of these cells. When they are appropriately stimulated by antigen present on macrophage membranes, proliferation and differentiation ensue.

   a. Small lymphocytes can also produce antibodies, but the major production is by the plasma cell.

   b. In most humoral immune responses, a second type of lymphocyte is also requisite. This **Th cell** acts synergistically with the plasma cell precursor to facilitate the production of mature antibody-forming cells. These are called **thymus-dependent humoral immune responses**.

   c. There are a few antigens that are able to induce antibody synthesis without the aid of Th cells; these are the **thymus-independent antigens**.

      (1) These antigens are usually carbohydrate [e.g., lipopolysaccharide (LPS) endotoxin], and are composed of monotonously repeating epitopes.

      (2) They induce IgM synthesis only and do not impart immunologic memory [i.e., no anamnestic response (see section IV A 3)].

IV. PHASES OF THE IMMUNE RESPONSE

A. Temporal phases

1. The **primary immune response** occurs following the first exposure to the antigen and is composed mainly of **IgM** antibody (Fig. 5-2).

2. Subsequent antigen exposures will cause the response to **shift to IgG production (IgM–IgG switch)**. This changeover appears to occur within individual plasma cells and is not the result of recruitment of new cells (IgG producers) to replace effete IgM-producing plasma cells.

3. If a sufficient length of time elapses after the primary antigenic stimulation, the antibody level will decrease markedly. However, a subsequent exposure to a small amount of antigen will evoke a rapid proliferation of plasma cells with the concomitant production of large amounts of specific antibody (see Fig. 5-2). This process, called an **anamnestic response** (also called **booster response, memory response,** or **secondary immune response**), occurs because a large population of antigen-reactive lymphocytes that are produced during the initial exposure to the antigen are recruited into the humoral immune response. These plasma cell precursors are called **memory cells** and represent another product of the collaboration between T cells and B cells (see section II D).

B. Ontogeny of the immune response. Adult levels of antibodies are not reached until the teenage years.

1. IgG is the major fetal antibody, and it is **acquired** from the mother through the placenta. IgM synthesis begins prior to birth and is the major antibody **produced** by a fetus. If IgM levels are elevated at birth, the infant may be infected.

2. The secretory IgA in colostrum provides local immunity for the infant in the intestinal tract, as well as providing protection for the mammary glands.

3. During the null period, several months after birth, the maternal IgG is being rapidly degraded and the infant has not yet begun to synthesize large quantities of IgG. This is the most dangerous time for an infant.

4. The development of full immunocompetence takes several years in humans and occurs in an ordered sequence that, in many ways, parallels the phylogenetic development of immune responses (Fig. 5-3).

V. CHARACTERISTICS OF THE CELLS INVOLVED IN THE IMMUNE RESPONSE are described below and are summarized in Table 5-1.

A. Macrophages are involved in both in vivo and in vitro immune responses, and have certain functional properties.

1. In the process of **phagocytosis**, macrophages function as effector cells as they recognize, engulf, and destroy foreign (antigenic) substances.

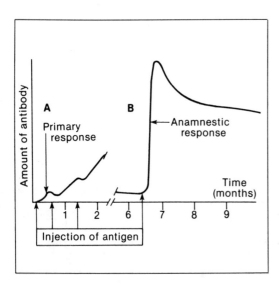

Figure 5-2. Phases of the humoral immune response. The time between initial and subsequent exposure to a specific antigen must be sufficient for an adequate immune response to be mounted. (*A*) A primary immune response occurs upon initial exposure; if the time between initial and subsequent antigen exposure is short, only a low-grade immune response is mounted. (*B*) If sufficient time elapses between exposures, an anamnestic response occurs, in which there is a rapid proliferation of plasma cells and production of a large amount of antibody specific for the antigen.

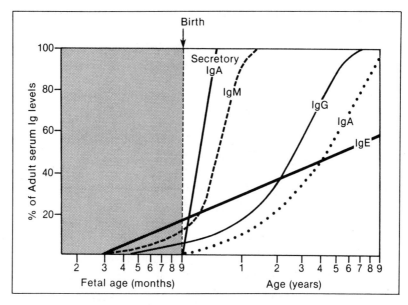

Figure 5-3. Development of immunocompetence with age in the human.

2. Macrophages are accessory cells in the immune response. They are the major **antigen-presenting cells** of the body that interact with antigen as a primary step in the **induction of an immune response**. B cells can also present antigen. Antigen presentation involves:
   a. **Binding and uptake of antigen** by the macrophage surface membrane, which creates a tightly bound antigen that is more immunogenic than free antigen
   b. **Processing and later reexpression of antigen** on the antigen-presenting cell surface in association with MHC (class II)-encoded glycoproteins
   c. **Release of soluble mediators**, such as the monokine (macrophage-derived hormone) **interleukin-1**, which stimulate the maturation and proliferation of T cells (the result of this sequence of events is the **activation of antigen-specific** B cells and T cells)

B. **Lymphocytes** are both precursor cells of immunologic function as well as regulators and effectors of immunity. Smaller lymphocytes (T cells) have a long life span of months or years, whereas larger lymphocytes (B cells) have a shorter life span of 5 to 7 days.

1. **A general method of detecting and quantitating T cells and B cells** depends on the differential reactivity of the two cell types with appropriately prepared red blood cells.

Table 5-1. Characteristics of Cells Involved in the Immune Response

Characteristics	T Cell	B Cell	Macrophage
Antigen-specific	+	+	−
Increased numbers in secondary response	+	+	−
Site of gamma globulin synthesis	−	+	−
Helper function in antibody response	+	−	−
Effector cell in cell-mediated immunity	+	−	−
Accessory cell in cell-mediated and humoral immunity	−	−	+
Antibody-binding receptors on surface	+	+ + +	−
Endotoxin receptor	−	+	−
Rosette with SRBC + antibody + component	−	+	−
Rosette with SRBC	+	−	−
Phytohemagglutinin receptor	+	−	−
Concanavalin A receptor	+	−	−
Lipopolysaccharide receptor	−	+	−

Note—SRBC = sheep red blood cells; + = characteristic of the cell; − = not a characteristic of the cell.

    a. T cells accumulate sheep red blood cells (SRBCs) around their surfaces and form clusters referred to as erythrocyte (E) rosettes.

    b. There is no such reaction between B cells and SRBCs, unless the red blood cells (indicated as **E** for erythrocytes) are coated with hemolysin [antibody (indicated as **A**)] and special nonhemolytic preparations of guinea pig complement (indicated as **C**), thus called **EAC rosettes.**

2. T cells

    a. Surface markers. T cells have antigen-specific receptors that function as antigen recognition sites and are the external expression of the cell's immunologic commitment (see section VI B). Surface antigens include **Thy 1**, **Lyt**, and differentiation antigens (e.g., T4, T8) identified by **monoclonal antibodies.**

       (1) In murine systems, the surface alloantigen called **theta** (*θ*), or **T antigen**, now referred to as two allelic forms, **Thy 1.1** and **Thy 1.2**, is acquired by lymphocytes as they enter and mature in the thymus. An analogous alloantigen exists on human T cells. Antiserum against this membrane marker is immunosuppressive and has been used to prevent rejection of transplanted tissue or organs.

       (2) Ly alloantigens also have been identified on murine T cells (**Lyt**) and B cells (**Lyb**). Lyt antigens have been useful in identifying functionally different subsets of mouse T cells.

       (3) Monoclonal antibody techniques have resulted in the differentiation of human T-cell maturation and functional T-cell subsets by the identification of various antigens on the cell membranes. These are identified by the prefix **T** (thymus) or **CD** (cellular differentiation).

          (a) T1, **T3**, and **T11** are found on most peripheral blood T cells. **T3** is associated with, but distinct from, the T-cell receptor for antigen; **T11**, with the SRBC rosette receptor.

          (b) T4 is present on Th cells, effector cells for delayed hypersensitivity, and Ts cell inducers.

          (c) T8 is present on cytotoxic and Ts cells.

          (d) T10 is present on stem cells, some B cells, and activated peripheral blood T cells.

    b. Thymic hormones are peptides that also **regulate the differentiation and maturation of T cells.** Thymic hormones include **thymosin**, **thymopoietin**, and **thymic humoral factor.**

    c. Mitogens. T cells have receptors for the plant lectins **phytohemagglutinin (PHA)** and **concanavalin A (ConA)**. When these receptors interact with the lectins, the cells are stimulated to divide (mitosis); hence, the stimulating molecules are called **mitogens**. ConA and PHA are considered to be T-cell–specific mitogens; however, **pokeweed mitogen (PWM)** stimulates mitosis in both T cells and B cells.

    d. Functions. Subpopulations of T cells have been defined according to the particular function of the subset, each of which demonstrates a particular activity exhibited by the entire T-cell population.

       (1) Effector T (Te) cells, also called T_{DTH} cells, are the peripheralized lymphocytic cells responsible for delayed type hypersensitivity (DTH) reactions.

       (2) Cytotoxic T (Tc) cells are induced artificially by immunization with allogeneic tissue and naturally by tumors and virus. To be induced to the killer function, the precursor cells must be stimulated by antigen in association with class II MHC molecules.

       (3) Memory T (Tm) cells are induced during primary immunization; they recognize the specific antigen and participate in the anamnestic response.

       (4) Helper T (Th) cells are lymphocytes that recognize a specific antigen in association with a homologous class II MHC molecule and collaborate with B cells and macrophages in the induction of the humoral immune response. Similar cells collaborate with other T cells to facilitate the production of Te cells.

       (5) Suppressor T (Ts) cells are lymphocytes that recognize a specific antigen and interfere with the development of an immune response either directly or via suppressor factors. These cells may be involved in the prevention of autoimmunity. Ts cell precursors are activated by antigens in association with a particular type of class II MHC molecule.

3. B cells

    a. Surface markers. Immunoglobulin is present as the primary surface marker on the B-cell membrane.

       (1) Surface immunoglobulin binds specific antigens and functions as an antigen recognition site that initiates the differentiation of the B cell, resulting in antibody synthesis. Contact between the antigen epitope and the immunoglobulin in the B-cell membrane triggers cell division. As this process continues, the B cell matures into a plasma cell with abundant rough endoplasmic reticulum, actively secreting large amounts of the antibody specifically reactive with its homologous epitope.

       (2) Other B-cell surface markers include histocompatibility antigens (HLA) in humans and

H-2 and Lyb alloantigens in murine B cells. HLA antigens are also on T cells and on most other nucleated cells of the body.

  b. Mitogens are responsible for stimulating the transformation of B cells into plasma cells. **Bacterial lipopolysaccharide (endotoxin)** is mitogenic for B cells only; hence, the relative proportions of B cells and T cells in a population can be estimated by using appropriate mitogens and measuring the uptake of radioactive thymidine (a precursor of DNA). PWM also stimulates B-cell mitosis.

  c. Function. B cells are divided into subpopulations according to the immunoglobulin class they synthesize (see Chapter 3, section III).

C. Non-B, non-T (null) lymphocytes are distinctly different from other lymphoid cells, particularly in their ability to express cytotoxicity prior to antigen exposure. **Natural killer (NK) cells** and **killer (K) cells** both exhibit this characteristic (see Chapter 1, section II E 1, 2).

VI. CELLULAR INTERACTIONS IN THE EXPRESSION AND REGULATION OF IMMUNITY

A. General considerations. The immune response requires cooperative interaction between distinct populations of immunocompetent cells. Both cell-mediated and humoral immunity are dependent on communication among populations of lymphocytes and macrophages. This communication involves recognition of three classes of immunologic determinants—MHC determinants, immunoglobulin idiotypes, and T-cell clonotypes.

B. The T-cell receptor for antigen. Antigen-induced activation of Tc cells, Te cells that participate in DTH, and Th cells requires that they "see" determinants of the antigen in the context of class II MHC determinants (see Chapter 12, section II B 3).

  1. The T-cell receptor for antigen consists of two polypeptide chains linked together by disulfide bonds; the chains have molecular weights of about 39,000 and 41,000. Both chains of the heterodimer are variable, although there may be more variability in the smaller chain.

  2. There is evidence that at least a portion of the T-cell receptor contains idiotypic determinants similar to those of immunoglobulin molecules.

  3. The heterodimer is noncovalently linked in the membrane to the T3 molecule. T3 appears late in differentiation when the cells are becoming immunocompetent. It is apparently not directly involved in antigen recognition, but antibodies against T3 spatially block the antigen-specific activation of T cells.

C. T-cell development. The ability of T cells to recognize self-MHC determinants is induced during their development in the thymus. T-cell differentiation in the thymus is also accompanied by the development of functional subpopulations of T cells that can be distinguished by differences in membrane display of certain differentiation antigens (see section V B 2 d).

D. T-cell activation

  1. Activation of Th and DTH-reactive T cells by antigen requires two signals, each of which is mediated by macrophages.

    a. The first signal requires the **presentation of antigen** in a manner suitable for recognition by T cells. Activation of Th and DTH-reactive T cells requires that they recognize antigen in conjunction with self Ia determinants (class II MHC-encoded cell membrane glycoproteins). Therefore, display of Ia determinants by macrophages is a prerequisite for antigen presentation. This requirement for MHC compatibility is referred to as **MHC restriction.**

    b. The second signal involves the synthesis and release of a soluble material termed **interleukin-1.**

      (1) Interleukin-1 appears to exert its effect by stimulating the production of a second distinct interleukin, **interleukin-2,** by T cells. Interleukin-2 then acts in concert with signals mediated by antigens plus Ia to allow full T-cell activation to proceed.

      (2) Interleukin-1 also has a positive effect on pre-B–cell maturation, as well as on clonal expansion of B cells following antigen stimulation.

  2. T cells interact with antigen presented in conjunction with Ia. This results in an increase in the expression of receptors for interleukin-2. Synthesis of interleukin-1 by accessory cells induces synthesis of interleukin-2 by the T cells, and it is the action of interleukin-2 that then allows full T-cell activation to proceed.

  3. The requirement of macrophages in the activation of Ts cells is different from that noted for the activation of Th and DTH-reactive T cells.

a. It has been suggested that in the absence of macrophage presentation, antigen is capable of directly activating Ts cells.

b. Whether or not activation of Ts cells requires liberation of a soluble material by accessory cells is not known.

c. It can be demonstrated that neither interleukin-1 nor interleukin-2 is sufficient to induce Ts cell activation.

4. Another interleukin, **interleukin-3**, has been shown to have potent growth-promoting activity for various hemopoietic cell lines and has been suggested as a requirement for the activation of Ts cells. Interleukin-3 has also been shown to induce **20-α-hydroxysteroid dehydrogenase**, a specific enzyme marker of mature T cells.

E. B-cell development

1. Two signals are required to induce the differentiation of B cells into antibody-secreting plasma cells.

   a. One signal is provided by interactions between antigen and B-cell immunoglobulin receptors.

   b. The second signal is mediated by Th cells; these latter signals require direct contact between T cells and B cells and are not mediated by soluble materials.

2. Soluble factors, broadly referred to as **B-cell growth factors**, are also involved in B-cell proliferation and maturation.

3. MHC restriction-T cells can only help B cells bearing identical class II Ia determinants.

VII. HYBRIDOMAS

A. General considerations. Hybridomas are artificially created cells that produce pure or monoclonal antibodies. Having a constant and uniform source of pure antibody, instead of the usual mixture produced by the immune system, not only affords a powerful research tool but can be expected to provide quicker and more accurate identification of viruses, bacteria, and cancer cells. The long-range promise of monoclonal antibodies is that they will be therapeutically useful as vaccine replacements and in the treatment of cancers.

B. The hybridoma technique

1. A mouse is injected with antigen and the antibody-making cells of its spleen are then fused in a test tube with a cancerous type of mouse cell known as a plasmacytoma, or myeloma, cell.

2. The hybrid cell so formed produces the single type of antibody molecule of its spleen cell parent and continually grows and divides, like its plasmacytoma cell parent.

3. Once the clone of cells producing the desired antibody has been selected, it can be grown as a continuous cell line from which large amounts of the pure or monoclonal antibody can be harvested.

4. Cells are cultured at high dilutions to allow only one fused cell per culture dish. **Only hybrid cells replicate** because plasma cells are end cells and the plasmacytoma cells employed are deficient in an enzyme (hypoxanthine-guanine phosphoribosyl transferase) which makes them susceptible to metabolic poisoning by appropriate alterations in the media.

5. The power of the method is that one or more specific antibodies can be developed against any organism or substance antigenic to the mouse. By contrast, the natural antibodies made against a given antigen are a mixed bag of molecules (i.e., a polyclonal antiserum), with each antibody targeted against a different epitope of the antigen.

6. The hybridoma technique produces mouse antibodies. However, these are not the first choice for therapy because of the body's reaction against foreign proteins. Efforts to develop the human equivalent of the mouse plasmacytoma cell should succeed within the next couple of years. An existing method of making human monoclonal antibodies is the **lymphoblastoid technique**. A human lymphocyte cell producing the desired antibody is transformed into a continuous cell line by being infected with Epstein-Barr virus. Unlike the hybridoma technique, where antibodies are raised against the antigen of choice, the lymphoblastoid technique requires screening human donors for the antibody needed.

STUDY QUESTIONS

Directions: Each question below contains five suggested answers. Choose the **one best** response to each question.

1. Most antibody is synthesized by the

(A) central lymphoid organs
(B) peripheral lymphoid organs
(C) primary lymphoid organs
(D) macrophages
(E) the Golgi apparatus

2. The monokine (macrophage-derived hormone) that is intimately involved in the immune response is

(A) interleukin-1
(B) interleukin-2
(C) interleukin-3
(D) macrophage-activating factor (MAF)
(E) migration-inhibiting factor (MIF)

3. The thymic lymphocytes that recognize an antigen and interfere with the development of a humoral immune response are called

(A) killer (K) cells
(B) helper T (Th) cells
(C) null cells
(D) contrasuppressor cells
(E) suppressor T (Ts) cells

4. Although T-cell and B-cell membranes contain some shared receptors, the receptor specific for B-cell membranes is

(A) pokeweed mitogen (PWM)
(B) phytohemagglutinin (PHA)
(C) concanavalin A (Con A)
(D) sheep red blood cells (SRBCs)
(E) C1q product of complement activation

Directions: Each question below contains four suggested answers of which **one or more** is correct. Choose the answer

A   if **1, 2, and 3** are correct
B   if **1 and 3** are correct
C   if **2 and 4** are correct
D   if **4** is correct
E   if **1, 2, 3, and 4** are correct

5. Which of the following characteristics describe the secondary (anamnestic) antibody response?

(1) Longer lag period after antigenic stimulus
(2) Greater absolute amount of antibody produced
(3) IgM production predominates
(4) A lower dose of immunogen is adequate to elicit the response

6. Cells with antigen-specific receptors include

(1) B cells
(2) helper T (Th) cells
(3) cytotoxic T (Tc) cells
(4) suppressor T (Ts) cells

7. Macrophages possess special properties and functions, including

(1) processing antigen
(2) production of interleukin-1
(3) presentation of antigen
(4) effecting the phagocytosis process

Directions: The group of questions below consists of lettered choices followed by several numbered items. For each numbered item select the **one** lettered choice with which it is **most** closely associated. Each lettered choice may be used once, more than once, or not at all.

Questions 8–14

For each cell characteristic or function, select the cell with which it is most closely associated.

(A) T cell
(B) B cell
(C) Macrophage
(D) Natural killer (NK) cell
(E) Neutrophil

8. Site of immunoglobulin synthesis

9. Helper function in antibody response

10. Suppressor cell

11. Rosettes only with sheep red blood cells (SRBCs) + antibody + complement (EAC)

12. Concanavalin A receptor

13. Phagocytizes an antigen and serves as a processing cell in the induction of immune responses

14. Expresses cytotoxicity prior to antigen exposure

ANSWERS AND EXPLANATIONS

1. The answer is B. (*II A 3*) Antibody synthesis occurs in peripheral lymphoid organs such as the tonsils, Peyer's patches, lymph nodes, and spleen. The central lymphoid organs, the thymus and the bursa of Fabricius or its mammalian counterpart, are the sites where lymphocytes receive their immunologic education and become committed to life as T or B cells.

2. The answer is A. (*V A 2 c*) Interleukin-1 is a product of the macrophage which it secretes during antigen processing. Interleukin-1 reacts with the helper T (Th) cell and induces it to produce interleukin-2. Interleukin-2 acts on other Th cells and causes their proliferation and elaboration of interleukin-3. Interleukin-3 causes the proliferation of many cells. Most important in the context of the immune response would be the proliferation of the B cell. Interleukin-1 is also known as endogenous pyrogen.

3. The answer is E. [*V B 2 d (5)*] Thymic suppressor (Ts) cells interfere with the development of humoral immune responses. Helper (Th) cells, on the other hand, are those which participate in an immune response in a positive manner. Both of these cells are of thymic origin. The helper cells release soluble mediators, or hormones, which enhance the immune response. Two of these are referred to as interleukin-2 and interleukin-3. These hormones induce the proliferation of other helper cells as well as B cells.

4. The answer is A. (*V B 3 b*) B-cell membranes contain receptors for pokeweed mitogen (PWM). When the PWM reacts with the B cell, it induces mitosis. This can be quantitated by measuring the amount of radioactive thymidine which is incorporated into the DNA of the cell. Pokeweed is also mitogenic for T cells, as is phytohemagglutinin (PHA) and concanavalin A (Con A). T cells also have in their membrane, a receptor for sheep erythrocytes. B cells contain a receptor for the C3b product of complement activation; they do not contain the receptor for C1q.

5. The answer is C (2, 4). (*IV A 3*) A characteristic of the secondary or anamnestic response is a more rapid production of antibody. In addition, there is a greater amount of antibody produced during this response. The antibody that predominates is IgG; IgM is characteristic of a primary immune response. It usually takes less immunogen to induce a secondary response than it does a primary response.

6. The answer is E (all). [*V B 2 d (2), (4), (5), 3 a (1)*] B cells contain epitope-specific receptors in their membrane, namely IgD and IgM (monomeric form) antibodies. Helper T (Th) cells, cytotoxic T (Tc) cells, and suppressor T (Ts) cells also have antigen specificity; therefore, they then also must have an antigen recognition mechanism. This is referred to as the T-cell receptor and has specificity for a particular epitope. The molecule has some homology with the Fab portion of immunoglobulin, but is not a partial antibody molecule.

7. The answer is E (all). (*V A 1, 2 a, b, c*) The macrophage is an antigen-processing cell. It presents the antigen to the specifically committed B cell and in the presence of the appropriate helper T (Th) cell, maturation and differentiation of the B cell occurs. Plasma cell progeny result from this maturational process. Macrophages also produce interleukin-1, a hormone which induces Th cell proliferation. Th cells release interleukin-2, which stimulates other Th cells to proliferate and, in addition, induces the production of interleukin-3, which causes proliferation of many different cells in the body, including B cells. Macrophages also function as effector cells in the phagocytosis process as they recognize, engulf, and destroy antigenic materials.

8–14. The answers are: 8-B, 9-A, 10-A, 11-B, 12-A, 13-C, 14-D. [*V A 2, B 1 b, 2 c, d (4), (5), 3 a (1), C*] Although most antibody is secreted by plasma cells, B cells also produce immunoglobulin and insert it into the membrane, where it is accessible to antigen. Interaction of the antigen on an accessory cell with its homologous cell-bound antibody will trigger lymphokine release and B-cell proliferation and differentiation if the cells are histocompatible at the class II major histocompatibility complex (MHC)-encoded protein. Helper T (Th) cells may also participate in this maturation to an antibody-secreting plasma cell; however, they also show MHC restriction.

There are several functional subsets of T cells. Th cells are important augmentors of B-cell maturation. They also function in cytotoxic T (Tc) cell development. The supressor T (Ts) cell has an opposing function; it serves to down-regulate (depress) the immune response. Helper T cells secrete interleukin-2 when appropriately stimulated by antigen and interleukin-1.

Suppressor cells are produced in the thymus and hence are T cells. They bear the T8 membrane antigen, as do Tc cells, and thus are easily distinguished from Th cells, which are OKT 8-, OKT 4+. Ts cells suppress directly, or via suppressor factors, the function of other immunologically active cells (e.g., helper cells). Precursors of Ts cells are activated by antigens in association with the class II MHC molecule.

T cells have receptors for sheep red blood cells (SRBCs) and hence will form rosettes when mixed with these cells. B cells will rosette with SRBCs if they are first coated with antibody and/or complement (specifically C3b). The phagocytic cells—macrophages, monocytes, and neutrophils—have receptors for C3b which act in the process of opsonization; these cells might also form rosettes with erythrocytes + antibody + complement (EAC) but they are eliminated from the assay prior to the addition of the C3b-bearing red blood cells.

Concanavalin A (Con A) is a T-cell–specific mitogen. It reacts with a receptor in the T-cell membrane and induces proliferation of these cells. Mitosis is quantitated by pulse-labeling the cells for 24 hours with tritiated thymidine.

Peripheral blood neutrophils are phagocytic. However, fixed macrophages such as the dendritic cells of the spleen and the Kupffer cells of the liver are also actively phagocytic, and are responsible for the initial phagocytosis of an antigen as it enters the spleen or lymph nodes. The processed antigen is presented to the lymphocytes on the macrophage membrane.

Natural killer (NK) cells are non-B, non-T (null) lymphocytes that are distinct in their ability to express cytotoxicity against targets (e.g., tumor cells, virally infected autologous cells, and transplanted tissues) in the absence of any previous exposure to the foreign materials. NK cells have a membrane receptor for the Fc portion of antibody but will kill targets in the absence of antibody.

6
Immune Regulation

I. INTRODUCTION. In clinical medicine, there are special instances when suppression or enhancement of immune responsiveness to selected antigens is desired.

    A. Management of immunodeficient patients involves the following general considerations.

        1. Avoidance of infection, if possible

        2. Vigorous use of antibiotics appropriate for the infectious agents involved

        3. Attempts at restoration of immune competence (e.g., through neutrophil infusion or administration of commercial gamma globulin)

        4. Attempts at reconstitution of immune competence (e.g., through fetal thymus or bone marrow transplantation)

    B. Responsiveness is the key to immune regulation.

        1. Unresponsiveness is the absence of an immune response to a substance that, under ordinary conditions, would be **immunogenic**. The substance has all the features necessary for antigenicity, but there is no immune response to it. Unresponsiveness can be divided into two broad categories: immunosuppression and tolerance. The difference between the two is primarily quantitative.

            a. Immunosuppression refers to a reduction in the host's entire immune responsiveness. Immunosuppression may be desirable under the following circumstances.

                (1) Allergic conditions of all sorts, both immediate and delayed hypersensitivities, can be handled by suppressing the immune response.

                (2) Autoimmune disease is so-called immunologic suicide where the body destroys its own tissues. Obviously, if normal tissues are being destroyed by an immune mechanism, the treatment is suppression of the immune response.

                (3) The rejection of grafted tissues and organs has an immunologic basis. Therefore, prolongation of graft survival can be enhanced by suppressing the patient's immune response.

            b. Tolerance is more restrictive and implies the absence of selected immune responses, thus producing a state of specific unresponsiveness (i.e., an immunotolerant state).

        2. Enhancement of responsiveness is referred to as **immunopotentiation**, and can be specific or nonspecific.

II. IMMUNOSUPPRESSION can occur by physical means, such as surgery and x-rays (γ-rays), and by chemical and biological actions.

    A. Physical immunosuppression

        1. Surgical manipulation can have a major impact on immune responsiveness.

            a. Two special types of **central lymphoid tissues** are the thymus and the bursa of Fabricius in birds, or certain **gut-associated lymphoid tissues (GALT)** or possibly bone marrow in mammals.

                (1) Surgical removal of the bursa, or the thymus, or both in the neonatal period will block the development of immunologic competence in the correspondingly dependent lymphoid cell line. It is necessary that these future antibody-producing cells receive some influence from the bursa before they can become responsive in peripheral lymphoid tissues. Similarly, it is necessary for small lymphocytes to differentiate in the thymus before they can function in peripheral tissue.

(2) Surgical removal of these tissues after immunologic development, however, has very little effect on immune competence, at least for a considerable period. Lymphoid cells require central lymphoid organ programming in order to differentiate appropriately in response to antigen in peripheral lymphoid tissues, but once that programming has been achieved, cells react as mature cells in peripheral tissues for months or years.

b. Removal of **peripheral lymphoid tissue** (e.g., the lymph nodes, spleen, and lymphoid cells in connective tissue) has little effect, because these tissues are too diffuse to be removed completely by surgical procedures. If they all could be removed, the animal would be completely immunologically unresponsive. Cells in lymph nodes and in the spleen percolate out and recirculate through the efferent lymphatics, which anastomose to form larger and larger collecting vessels, and finally the fluid and cells of the efferent lymphatics become part of the thoracic duct. When the thoracic duct is cannulated and the lymphoid cells are removed, a very severe immunologic deficiency is produced.

2. Radiation acts on the lymphoid cells and bone marrow. Shielding the lymphoid organs from irradiation protects against diminished immune capacity.

a. X-rays produce various immunosuppressive effects on the primary immune response.

(1) Radiation damages DNA; thus, cells that are in the process of division or that need to divide to express their immunologic role will be most affected by this exposure.

(2) Once antigen interacts with an immunologically committed lymphocyte, it triggers cell division with concomitant differentiation and maturation into plasma cells or specifically sensitized cytotoxic T cells.

b. The secondary immune response is affected very slightly by x-rays, because the cells involved do not require DNA synthesis (i.e., they do not need to divide).

B. Chemical and biological immunosuppressive agents include therapeutic agents for autoimmune disease, some of which are also cancer chemotherapeutics. Most anticancer agents have some degree of immunosuppressive activity.

1. General considerations

a. All chemical and biological immunosuppressive agents are more effective in preventing a primary immune response than they are in preventing a secondary immune response or in interrupting an ongoing response.

(1) In order to block responsiveness, it is important that the immunosuppressive agent be given for some time before the antigen. For example, kidney transplant patients are started on immunosuppressive therapy before the transplant operation.

(2) Once the patient has started to respond, the injection of immunosuppressive agents is much less effective.

b. Immunosuppressive drugs are more effective in preventing homograft rejecton than they are in treating allergies or autoimmune diseases. In the latter two cases, the disorder is diagnosed by the presence of antibody or sensitized lymphoid cells in the patient's tissues; hence, the immune response has already been induced.

c. Since a role of the immune response is limitation or protection against infectious disease, the result of immunosuppression with any of these drugs or with any other procedure is increased incidence and chronicity of infectious disease. When immunosuppressive agents are used, the patient is more subject to infectious disease and malignancy.

2. Action of immunosuppressive agents

a. Lympholytic agents can block the expression of the immune response (through cell lysis) but still are more effective in blocking the initiation of the immune response. The two major types of lympholytic immunosuppressants are **ionizing radiation** and **antiserum** (i.e., antilymphocyte serum and antithymocyte serum). Both types are effective against cell-mediated immunity and block both the induction of an immune response and the expression of one already induced. These are used in situations such as renal and cardiac transplantation.

b. Lymphocytotoxic agents interfere with metabolic processes (usually DNA synthesis) of lymphocytes in such a manner as to block cell division or otherwise interrupt vital cell functions such as RNA or protein synthesis. They are most efficient at interrupting the inductive phase of an immune response.

(1) Antimetabolites, such as purine and pyrimidine analogs and folic acid antagonists (methotrexate), interfere with DNA synthesis.

(2) Alkylating agents, such as cyclophosphamide, interfere with cell division by altering guanine so that base pairing errors occur. They also can cross-link the two strands, thus blocking DNA replication.

(3) Antibiotics, such as cyclosporine, exert an inhibitory effect on interleukin-2 action, thus blocking the expansion of the helper/inducer T-cell population. It is particularly effective in suppressing graft rejection reactions.

(4) **Cortisone** is immunosuppressive as well as anti-inflammatory. In laboratory animals it is lympholytic, but not in humans, where it seems to alter cell migration and cause lymphopenia and monocytopenia shortly after injection. Cortisone has the following effects.

(a) It depresses macrophage chemotaxis and interleukin-1 production.

(b) It inhibits calcium ion influx into cells.

(c) It depresses release and/or effect of interleukin-2, lymphotoxin, macrophage migration-inhibition factor (MIF), and macrophage-activating factor (MAF).

(d) It blocks cleavage of membrane phospholipids, thus lowering prostaglandin and leukotriene levels by inhibiting arachadonic acid release from the membrane.

c. **Antibodies** are used to inhibit immune responses in three ways.

(1) Antibodies that react with lymphoid cells, such as antilymphocyte globulins or antilymphocyte serum, are used. Because there are two types of lymphoid cells (i.e., the T cells and B cells), antilymphocyte sera can be produced that will react more or less specifically with one or the other.

(a) If injected into the body, the antibodies against T cells can find all the lymphocytes in the lymph nodes, blood, and other components of the reticuloendothelial system. This is the means of attacking peripheral lymphoid tissue to produce wanted immunosuppression.

(b) Antilymphocyte serum, particularly antithymocyte serum, is most useful in inducing immune deficiency in transplant patients by suppression of all cell-mediated immune responses (see Chapter 12, section V A 4).

(2) If a preformed antibody is injected into an animal, followed by injection of specific antigen, the immune response in the host will be blocked. The injected antibody binds up the antigen and prevents its access to lymphoid tissue. This is the principle through which $Rh_0(D)$ immunoglobulin (**RhoGAM**) was developed to combat Rh incompatibility (**erythroblastosis fetalis**). Antiserum against the immunogen (Rh antigen) will neutralize the antigen through some mechanism (probably by coating it in such a way that it is cleared from the body very rapidly); thus, an immune response is aborted.

(3) If antibodies that are specific for the antigen-combining site (the idiotype) of an antibody are injected into an animal, they can specifically abort that particular immune response. This anti-idiotype–induced unresponsive state is really a case of immune tolerance (see section III B), as only one specific immune response is affected.

C. **Immunosuppression associated with diseases.** A reduction of immune competence may accompany various disease states. This is usually due to a direct effect on the immune apparatus itself (see Chapter 11), but it may also occur as a side effect of the primary disease.

1. **Congenital immunodeficiencies**

   a. **Bruton's hypogammaglobulinemia** is characterized by a failure of development of B-cell (humoral) immunity. These patients form antibodies very poorly and suffer from repeated bacterial infections (see Chapter 11, section III A).

   b. **DiGeorge syndrome** occurs due to failure of development of the third and fourth pharyngeal pouches during embryogenesis. These patients have a great deal of trouble with recurrent viral diseases (see Chapter 11, section IV A).

2. **Malignancies** are potentially immunosuppressive, particularly if they involve lymphoid tissues. Lymphomas (e.g., Hodgkin's disease and sarcoidosis) may disrupt normal lymphocyte functions directly or may "crowd out" normal lymphocytes from bone marrow and peripheral lymphoid tissues.

3. **Infections** can also induce immunosuppression.

   a. Measles and certain other viral diseases cause a transient depression in cell-mediated immune responses.

   b. Human T-cell lymphotropic virus [(HTLV-III), also known as human immunodeficiency virus (HIV)] infection causes a profound immunosuppression which renders the host susceptible to fatal infections caused by opportunistic pathogens.

   c. Specific energy is seen in lepromatous leprosy and the terminal stages of tuberculosis.

4. **Malnutrition** is a major cause of immunodeficiency.

   a. Adequate nutrition is essential for proper functioning of the immune system. Cell-mediated immunity appears to be the most sensitive to nutritional deprivation, but humoral immunity, complement, and phagocytic functions are also affected.

   b. Nutrient deficiencies that adversely affect immune functions include:

   (1) Protein deficiency

(2) Vitamin deficiencies, particularly those involved in DNA and protein synthesis (e.g., A, B_6, B_{12}, and folic acid)

(3) Mineral deficiencies, particularly zinc and iron, which can cause decreases in T-cell functions and microbicidal activity of phagocytes

III. TOLERANCE is the absence of specific immune responses in an otherwise fully immunocompetent person. This type of unresponsiveness can be either naturally acquired (**autotolerance**) or specifically induced (**acquired** or **immune tolerance**). Escape from the former may result in autoimmune diseases, while induction of the latter could represent an avenue for therapy of these diseases, as well as allergic conditions and allograft rejection.

A. Autotolerance, also called **neonatal** or **natural tolerance**, is acquired early in life.

1. Animals probably acquire autotolerance in utero. During fetal development, the ability to recognize one's own tissues is acquired. From that point, individuals do not ordinarily produce antibodies against their own normal tissue antigens (**self antigens**).

2. There are many theories as to why autotolerance exists, but the most favored is referred to as the **clonal deletion theory**.
   a. A clone is the progeny of a single cell. It is probable that clones of cells capable of responding to an individual's own tissues arise throughout life. These clones are called **forbidden clones** and are immediately deleted by encountering an overwhelming amount of self antigens or by the activity of antigen-specific suppressor cells.
   b. Very often this suppression (i.e., autotolerance) works less effectively than it should, the result being **autoimmune disease**.

B. Immune tolerance. Autotolerance can be simulated by a very simple experiment. However, because the procedure is contrived and the unresponsive state is not natural, the phenomenon is called acquired or immune tolerance.

1. A host (e.g., a fetal animal) can be induced into unresponsiveness by the injection of a foreign substance (thus mimicking the autoantigen exposure that induces autotolerance). The animal will assume that the substance is self antigen, and it will not produce an antibody response to that substance later in life.

2. The only way to perpetuate this unresponsiveness is to maintain continually a low level of that antigen in the animal. The mechanism is probably the same as when this happens spontaneously or naturally.

3. Immune tolerance is usually induced by excessive amounts of antigen. The mechanism is probably quite similar to that of autotolerance; that is, the antibody-producing cells or the cells capable of mounting a response are overwhelmed and deleted. The large dose of antigen that will induce tolerance is referred to as the **tolerogenic dose**.

4. The antibody-producing cells are antigen-reactive or antigen-sensitive cells. **Tolerance** is not simply in vivo neutralization or absorption of the antibody—it **is the specific absence of antibody-forming cells induced by tolerogen**.

5. It is possible to have gradations of tolerance.
   a. In **partial tolerance**, the individual is unable to respond to some of the epitopes on the antigen but can respond to others.
   b. Immune deviation, also known as **split tolerance**, is the state where one of the immune responses can be interfered with, but not another. For example, the IgM response may be blocked, but not the IgG response. Alternately, the cell-mediated response may be blocked, but not the humoral response.

6. **Tolerance is a specific cellular defect** that is probably due to the absence of a cell. This may involve two of the three cells in the immune response. The macrophage does not have specificity, so it cannot be directly involved in tolerance. The T cells and B cells have specificity, so they can be involved. The role of the T cell and the B cell has been extensively investigated in mice.
   a. It has been found that T-cell tolerance will occur 1 day after the tolerogen is given and will last 120–150 days.
   b. In contrast, it will take 5–7 days for the B cell to become tolerant, and this will last for only about 50 days.
   c. Further, it requires only 1/1000 the amount of antigen to induce T-cell tolerance as opposed to B-cell tolerance.

7. **Tolerance is antigen-specific.** The unresponsiveness is to the one antigen and all or only some of its epitopes.

a. Cross-reacting antigens can break tolerance to some epitopes if two conditions are met.
   (1) The immunogen contains new epitopes plus a common (shared) one to which the animal is unresponsive.
   (2) The unresponsiveness is in the T-cell compartment only; that is, epitope-specific B cells must be available to be "triggered" to differentiate into plasma cells.
b. When the immunogen is injected, it will recruit a helper T cell reactive with the new epitope and cooperation of this cell with the B cell [spared because of condition (2)] will ensue.

8. There are several factors that influence tolerance induction.
   a. Immune tolerance (in either the T cell or B cell) is easier to induce in the neonate or the prenatal animal. It then follows that as the ease of induction is greatest with the least immunologic maturity, immunosuppression enhances tolerance induction.
   b. The simpler the antigen, the better tolerogen it will be. The more complex it is, the less effective it will be in inducing tolerance. Thus, bacterial and mammalian cells are extremely poor tolerogens. This is probably related to the high density of different epitopes as well as to their propensity for phagocyte interaction, an event that seems to drive the immune response forward in a positive direction.
   c. A **threshold** amount of antigen is required to induce tolerance. An increase over this amount may increase the duration of tolerance but will not hasten its onset. The longer a tolerogen can persist in an animal above the threshold, the longer the duration of tolerance will be.

9. The following methods are employed in the induction of immune tolerance.
   a. Adult animals are usually immunosuppressed by injection of cyclosporine or another suitable agent, or they are injected with a tolerogenic form of the antigen. For example, a saline solution of human gamma globulin would normally be immunogenic, but if the aggregated forms of the antigen are removed by ultracentrifugation, the solution becomes tolerogenic.
   b. The antigen can be complexed with a toxic compound such as ricin or daunomycin, or labeled with a radioactive isotope such as iodine-125. The B cells and T cells bearing membrane receptors for the antigen can thus be destroyed, eliminating that specific immune reactivity.
   c. Anti-idiotype cytotoxic antibody can be injected to eliminate a specific clone of B cells. Similarly, an animal could be treated with an antiserum specific for the epitope-reactive portion of the T-cell antigen receptor (a clonotypic antibody), thus blocking cell-mediated immune responses.

10. There are two theories of how immune tolerance is induced. Both of these mechanisms are probably operative in nature. Figure 6-1 shows a schematic representation of the mechanisms of tolerance induction.

    a. One theory states that the B cell, which will form the plasma cell, is rendered tolerant by an antigen blockade at the membrane. The B cell has specific membrane receptors for antigen and tolerogen. When these receptors react with tolerogen, they are fixed, or frozen, such that no messages for antibody production can get into the cell. The cells may, in fact, be killed by interaction with the tolerogen. Tolerance in the thymus cell may have a similar mechanism.
    b. An alternate theory states that tolerogen induces the generation of specific suppressor cells. These cells interact directly with helper T cells or plasma cell precursors to block their maturation. In addition, antigen-specific or nonspecific soluble immune response suppressive factors have been isolated from T cells.

IV. **IMMUNOPOTENTIATION.** Enhancement of the immune response can be affected by increasing the rate at which the response occurs, elevating its magnitude, prolonging the response, or directing the response to a particular facet of the immune response. Substances capable of these actions may be specific or nonspecific potentiators.

A. **Nonspecific potentiators** are called **adjuvants**. Adjuvants are substances that enhance the immunogenicity of molecules without altering their chemical composition. Adjuvants enhance immune responses by their ability to increase the efficiency of macrophage processing of antigen, prolong the period of exposure to the antigen, and amplify the proliferation of immunologically committed lymphocytes. A list of representative adjuvants and their possible mechanism of action is presented in Table 6-1.

   1. **Freund's adjuvant** is a classic adjuvant that is an emulsion of paraffin or mineral oil (usually Bayol F) and water. Lanolin and arlacel A are used as emulsifying agents.

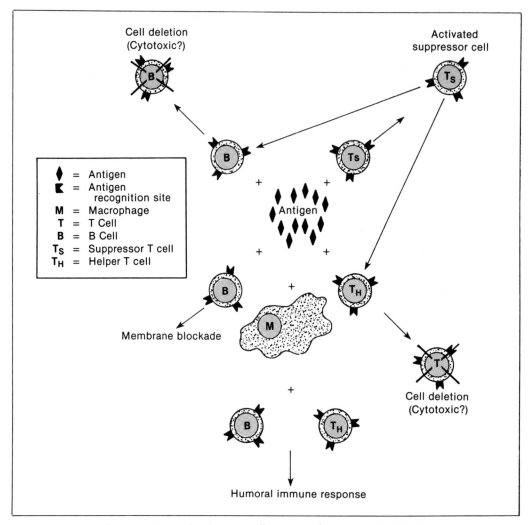

Figure 6-1. Potential pathways to effect immunologic nonresponsiveness.

    a. Incomplete Freund's adjuvant (IFA) is a water-in-oil emulsion with antigen in the water phase. It will increase the humoral immune response about 100-fold, greatly reduce the amount of antigen required (10 μ will immunize a rabbit), and prolong the phase of active immunoglobulin synthesis by months.

    b. If mycobacteria or cell wall components of these organisms are added, the product is called **complete Freund's adjuvant (CFA)**. The addition of the bacteria does not markedly enhance the antibody response but it does add another dimension to the response—the response of the host will include cell-mediated immunity as well as antibody synthesis. Thus, if an antigen like ovalbumin is injected with CFA, the animal will develop high levels of circulating antibody as well as a strong T-cell response to ovalbumin.

2. Aluminum hydroxide and **alum** have a mechanism of action similar to Freund's adjuvant in retarding absorption of the antigen and thus prolonging exposure to antibody-forming tissues. They also will cause local inflammation, thus increasing mononuclear cell exposure.

3. Another example of a directional influence of an adjuvant is the elevated IgE response seen when heat-killed ***Bordetella pertussis*** organisms are present in a vaccine.

4. Lymphokines, such as interleukin-1, -2, and -3 and interferon, enhance lymphocyte proliferation and activate immunocompetent lymphoid cells.

5. Mitogenic substances, such as endotoxin, produce an immunostimulatory effect by increasing the clonal expansion of B cells and T cells.

Table 6-1. Classification of Immunopotentiator Compounds

Class	Mechanism	Compound
Depot Water-in-oil emulsion	Delayed release of antigen; prolongation of lymphoid tissue exposure to antigen	Freund's adjuvant
Precipitants and absorbents		Calcium alginate Alum Aluminum hydroxide Bentonite Polyacrylamide Methylated bovine serum albumin
Irritant	Induce chronic inflammatory response which increases antigen exposure to macrophages and B cells and T cells	The substances listed above are foreign bodies and will induce an inflammatory response. Mycobacteria, especially wax D and muramyl dipeptide of the cell wall
Mitogenic	Increase clonal expansion of B cells and T cells during an immune response	Lipopolysaccharide (endotoxin) of gram-negative bacteria Phytohemagglutinin Concanavalin A
Lymphokines	Enhance proliferation and/or differentiatin of lymphoid cells; activate macrophages	Interleukin-1, -2, and -3 Macrophage activating factor Interferons
Synthetic polynucleotides	Stimulate antigen processing and helper T-cell activity	Polyadenylate-uridylate

6. **Corynebacterium parvum** is a gram-positive rod that has been used as an experimental immunotherapeutic agent in cancer patients. Heat-killed, formaldehyde-treated cell vaccines activate macrophages, which display increased phagocytosis and cytotoxicity.

7. **Bacille Calmette-Guérin (BCG)** is a well-studied immune potentiator. It is an attenuated tubercle bacillus that is used as a vaccine against tuberculosis. It causes macrophage activation and also enhances natural killer cell activity.

B. **Specific potentiators.** There are some factors that have immunologic specificity.

1. **Helper factors** are secreted by T cells following interaction of their antigen-specific receptor with its homologous epitope.

2. **Transfer factor** is an antigen-specific dialyzable extract of immune T cells that is capable of transferring cell-mediated immunity.

3. An **immunogenic RNA** has been extracted from lymphoid tissues of experimental animals following antigen injection. This appears to be an antigen epitope complexed with cellular RNA which greatly increases the immunogenicity of the molecule.

STUDY QUESTIONS

Directions: Each question below contains five suggested answers. Choose the **one best** response to each question.

1. The injection of large doses of protein results in immune tolerance that appears to be due to

(A) removal of antibody by excess antigen
(B) catabolism of antibody as rapidly as it is formed
(C) production of a nonreacting antibody
(D) suppression of B-cell or T-cell differentiation, proliferation, or both
(E) induction of cytotoxic anti-idiotype antibodies

2. The immunosuppressive effect of cortisone is attributed to its ability to

(A) produce lymphopenia
(B) destroy immunoglobulins
(C) block DNA synthesis
(D) stabilize lysosomal membranes
(E) cross-link DNA strands

3. Erythroblastosis fetalis can be prevented if the mother is injected, at parturition, with an antibody called

(A) blocking antibody
(B) Rh$_0$(D) immunoglobulin (RhoGAM)
(C) antilymphocyte globulin
(D) antithymocyte serum
(E) univalent antiserum

4. Which of the following adjuvants will induce an increase in the IgE response?

(A) Incomplete Freund's adjuvant
(B) Complete Freund's adjuvant
(C) *Bordetella pertussis*
(D) *Corynebacterium parvum*
(E) Alum

5. A serious complication of the use of immunosuppressive agents is the

(A) increased incidence of autoimmune diseases
(B) loss of tuberculin sensitivity in tuberculosis patients
(C) increased susceptibility to opportunistic infections
(D) loss of hair
(E) decrease in complement levels

6. Lympholytic immunosuppressive agents include

(A) cortisone
(B) actinomycin D
(C) x-rays
(D) cyclosporine
(E) methotrexate

Directions: Each question below contains four suggested answers of which **one or more** is correct. Choose the answer

A if **1, 2, and 3** are correct
B if **1 and 3** are correct
C if **2 and 4** are correct
D if **4** is correct
E if **1, 2, 3, and 4** are correct

7. If the emergence of forbidden clones is not continuously suppressed throughout life, a person may develop

(1) hypergammaglobulinemia
(2) allergic conditions
(3) autotolerance
(4) autoimmune disease

8. Patients receiving long-term immunosuppression commonly experience

(1) recurrence of herpes simplex and other viral infections
(2) decrease in antibody synthesis
(3) loss of T-cell immunity
(4) loss of suppressor T cells

9.   Immunosuppressive measures are most effective when administered

(1) just prior to antigen exposure
(2) 1 week before antigen exposure
(3) at the time of antigen exposure
(4) following antigen exposure

10. Immunopotentiating compounds that act as antigen depots include

(1) alum
(2) polyadenylate-uridylate
(3) aluminum hydroxide
(4) interferon

11. Bacterial products that enhance the immune response include

(1) lymphokine
(2) immunogenic RNA
(3) transfer factor
(4) endotoxin

ANSWERS AND EXPLANATIONS

1. The answer is D. [*III B 3, 6, 7 a (2)*] Large doses of antigen induce immune tolerance by eliminating helper T cells and specifically reactive B cells. In most experimental systems, circulating antibody would not be present prior to tolerogen administration. In fact, free antibody can interfere with tolerance induction. Cytotoxic anti-idiotype antibodies can induce immune tolerance, but their production would not be induced by injection of the antigen.

2. The answer is A. [*II B 2 b (4)*] Cortisone produces lymphopenia, either by direct lympholytic action, as seen in rodents, or by altering the tissue distribution of these cells in humans. T cells are more sensitive than B cells to the effect of corticosteroids. These drugs also have an anti-inflammatory action and interfere with lysosomal membrane fusion with phagosomes.

3. The answer is B. [*II B 2 c (2)*] $Rh_0(D)$ immunoglobulin (RhoGAM) reacts with fetal erythrocytes in the mother's circulation and opsonizes them. They are phagocytized by the reticuloendothelial system and destroyed before they can induce an immune response. RhoGAM cannot interfere with a secondary response to the D (Rh) antigen; therefore, it must be used in the first pregnancy. It is a blocking agent, not a means of inducing immune tolerance to the D antigen; hence, it should be administered at the end of each pregnancy.

4. The answer is C. (*IV A 3*) *Bordetella pertussis* has an adjuvant action that induces the production of IgE antibodies in experimental animals. Freund's adjuvants (either complete or incomplete) are water and oil emulsions in which the antigen is emulsified in the oil phase. Complete Freund's adjuvant has mycobacteria or mycobacterial cell products incorporated into the emulsion. Both of these adjuvants are used in experimental situations, but are not used in humans. They function, as does alum, by being an irritant, causing an inflammatory response at the site of adjuvant deposition, and by serving as a depot from which antigen is slowly released to the antibody-forming system of the body. *Corynebacterium parvum* is an adjuvant that enhances macrophage activity.

5. The answer is C. (*II B 1 c*) Drug-induced immunodeficiency commonly increases the incidence of infections, particularly by opportunistic pathogens. Cancer frequency also is higher in individuals receiving immunosuppressive therapy. Tuberculin sensitivity would probably not be affected as immunosuppression is not very effective against established responses. Hair loss is a common complication of cancer chemotherapy, but the dosages of drugs used in control of autoimmune diseases, graft rejection episodes, and so forth usually is not high enough to manifest this unpleasant side effect.

6. The answer is C. (*II B 2 a*) Lysis of lymphoid cells can be caused by ionizing radiation and specific antibodies to appropriate cell membrane markers. Cortisone causes lympholysis in some animal species but not in humans. Here its action is more directed to changing the traffic pattern of the cells. Actinomycin D, cyclosporine, and methotrexate interfere with DNA replication or function and hence cause immunosuppression.

7. The answer is D (4). (*III A 2 a, b*) One of the theories of the origin of autoimmunity hypothesizes that the disease is due to the emergence of clones of cells (forbidden clones) that are autoreactive. These clones are triggered to proliferate and mature into immunologically competent effector cells that attack self antigen by contact with cross-reactive antigens or altered native molecules. Another theory suggests that B cells reactive with self antigen are present naturally and their development into plasma cells secreting autoantibodies occurs because a helper T cell has been recruited by a second epitope on the immunogen.

8. The answer is E (all). (*I B 1 a; II B 1 c*) Patients suffering from autoimmune disease, or individuals bearing transplants that require immunosuppression, commonly suffer from recurrent herpes simplex infections, as well as other manifestations of viral disease. They will have a decrease in total antibody synthesis and will have depression of cell-mediated immune responses. Both cytotoxic and suppressor T cells may be depressed in individuals under long-term immunosuppression.

9. The answer is B (1, 3). (*II B 1 a*) Immunosuppressive therapy is usually directed at cells in the process of proliferation and hence is most effective if given just before, or at the time of, antigen administration. It is far more difficult to block ongoing responses and booster responses because the need for proliferation is not as marked. If the suppression occurs too far in advance of the immunization, the drug effect will have worn off.

10. The answer is B (1, 3). (*IV A 2; Table 6-1*) Alum-coprecipitated and aluminum hydroxide-adsorbed antigen retard absorption from the site of injection. In this manner they extend the period of antigen exposure. They also are irritants and increase macrophage and lymphoid cell exposure to the antigen. Polyadenylate-uridylate stimulates macrophage processing of antigens and also enhances helper T cell activity. Interferons are products of various cells of the body which increase proliferation and maturation of lymphoid cells. They also activate macrophages

11. The answer is D (4). *(IV A 4, 5, B 2, 3)* Endotoxin, the lipopolysaccharide component of the cell wall of most gram-negative bacteria, is immunopotentiating by virtue of its ability to induce proliferation in B cells. It acts as a polyclonal activator and can nonspecifically trigger humoral immune responses. Lymphokines are products of lymphocytes which have a positive effect on the immune response. Transfer factor is a soluble mediator of delayed hypersensitivity; that is, it is released by specifically sensitized T cells and can confer identical reactivity to naive T cells. Immunogenic RNA is primarily a laboratory phenomenon wherein RNA extracted from lymphoid tissues of immunized animals will exhibit enhanced immunogenicity in a second experimental animal.

7
Immunization

I. INTRODUCTION. The practice of immunization began in antiquity with the realization that individuals who recovered from certain diseases were often protected against recurrence of the same illness.

    A. In 1798, Edward Jenner introduced the use of vaccination with cowpox to protect individuals against smallpox. This contribution, followed some years later by the observation by Louis Pasteur that attenuated rabies virus would protect individuals against rabies, ushered in a modern era devoted to the search for immunizing agents that would, with a minimum of risk to the host, provide long-term protection against infectious disease.

    B. Agents used for immunization can be administered by several routes and can be divided into vaccines used for active immunization (immunoprophylaxis) and serum preparations (antitoxin, immune globulin, and specific immune globulin) used for passive immunization (immunotherapy).

II. ROUTES OF ADMINISTRATION

    A. Injection is the most common method used for immunization. Several injection routes are available.

        1. Intramuscular and **subcutaneous injections** are the methods used most often.

        2. Intradermal (intracutaneous) injection is often used for revaccination of previously inoculated individuals.

    B. Oral administration came into widespread use with the introduction of the Sabin polio vaccine, a live attenuated virus preparation that multiplies and infects and immunizes the recipient. In the process, vaccine virus is disseminated in the community.

    C. Intranasal administration has gained interest, stimulated by the finding that, in upper respiratory disease, natural infection results in the production of specific antibodies both in serum and in secretions at the local site of infection. Intranasal immunization should stimulate an immune response that mimics the response induced by natural infection. The procedure is currently being evaluated with influenza vaccination.

III. ACTIVE IMMUNIZATION (IMMUNOPROPHYLAXIS). Active, artificially acquired immunity is induced by the administration of vaccines which consist of either intact microorganisms (killed or attenuated) or their component parts or products that are unable to produce disease but are still antigenic and able to induce an immune response (see Chapter 1, section I B 1; Table 1-1).

    A. Bacterial vaccines

        1. Intact bacteria used for immunization may be either dead or living.
            a. For the preparation of **dead bacterial vaccines**, the organisms are cultured, harvested after suitable incubation, and then killed with heat or chemicals (e.g., acetone, formalin, thimerosal, phenol). Killing must be designed to preserve the immunogenicity of the preparation.
            b. Live attenuated (weakened) bacterial vaccines can be prepared by frequent subculture on artificial media. Live attenuated agents are generally preferable because they provide a superior and long-lived immune response.

2. Bacterial products used for immunization are usually either **structural components** or **detoxified products (toxoids)**.

    a. The capsule of certain bacteria (e.g., *Streptococcus pneumoniae*) is an example of a structural component that has proved to be valuable in vaccination. It induces the production of anticapsular antibodies that neutralize the antiphagocytic effect of the capsule. M protein (group A streptococcus) and pili (*Neisseria gonorrhoeae*) are other examples of structural components of value in immunization.

    b. Toxins can be converted into nontoxic but still immunogenic preparations called **toxoids**. Heat or formalin can be used for their preparation. The resulting material is called **natural fluid plain toxoid**, which induces the production of antitoxic antibody. Adjuvants are sometimes used to prolong the antigenic stimulus.

        (1) Alum-precipitated toxoid is toxoid that has been precipitated by the addition of potassium aluminum sulfate, then washed, and suspended in saline.

        (2) Adsorbed toxoid is toxoid that has been adsorbed onto particles of aluminum hydroxide or aluminum phosphate.

3. Representative currently used vaccines

    a. Diphtheria toxoid is available as a fluid toxoid of *Corynebacterium diphtheriae*, but is more immunogenic when precipitated with potassium alum or adsorbed onto aluminum hydroxide or aluminum phosphate. It is commonly combined with tetanus toxoid and pertussis vaccine as **DPT vaccine**.

    b. Pertussis vaccine is administered for whooping cough vaccination. It consists of a thimerosal-killed or heat-killed preparation of *Bordetella pertussis* organisms. Only bacteria in a capsule form can be used for this vaccine, since the presence of a capsule correlates with virulence.

    c. Tetanus toxoid is a preparation of inactivated *Clostridium tetani* toxin. It is available as fluid toxoid but it is most immunogenic when adsorbed.

    d. Bacille Calmette-Guérin (BCG) vaccine is a live attenuated strain (see section III B 1) of *Mycobacterium bovis* that is used as a vaccination against **tuberculosis**.

    e. Typhoid vaccine is a suspension of heat- or acetone-killed *Salmonella typhi* that is effective against typhoid fever.

    f. Pneumococcal polysaccharide vaccine was originally prepared from the polysaccharide capsule of 14 antigenically different strains of *S. pneumoniae*. A pool containing capsular material from 23 antigenic types of organisms is currently available to provide immunity against bacteremic pneumococcal disease.

    g. *Haemophilus influenzae* vaccine is prepared from the polysaccharide capsule of *H. influenzae* type b to provide immunity against bacterial meningitis.

B. Viral and rickettsial vaccines

1. Live attenuated viral vaccines have the advantage of mimicking natural infection. They multiply in the vaccinated host and stimulate long-lasting antibody production. It should be emphasized, however, that they carry the risk of reversion to virulence. Attenuation can be accomplished by repeated subculture in tissue culture or by serial passage in various animal hosts.

2. Killed (inactivated) preparations are safer, in general, but the immunity conferred is often brief and must be boosted. Inactivation can be accomplished with formalin or ultraviolet light.

3. Representative currently used vaccines

    a. Viral

        (1) Rubella (German measles) vaccine contains live attenuated virus grown in tissue culture (e.g., rabbit kidney, duck embryo, and human diploid cells). The preferred culture is human diploid cells.

        (2) Influenza virus vaccine consists of whole virus or disrupted (split) virus products grown in chick embryo and inactivated by formalin or ultraviolet light. Composition of the vaccine varies depending on epidemiologic circumstances.

            (a) Of the three serotypes of influenza virus, only influenza types a and b are involved in human influenza vaccine.

            (b) However, new antigenic subtypes continually evolve. To compensate for the frequent **antigenic shift** of the influenza virus, new vaccines that will be effective against new strains need to be developed.

        (3) Measles and **mumps vaccines** are live attenuated viruses grown in chick embryos.

        (4) Poliomyelitis vaccine is currently available in two forms.

            (a) Salk vaccine, also called **inactivated polio vaccine (IPV)**, is a virus grown in tissue culture (e.g., monkey kidney) that is inactivated with formalin or ultraviolet light.

This form of the vaccine is administered intramuscularly and provides immunity from paralytic or systemic disease but not against polio virus infection.

    (b) Sabin vaccine is a live attenuated **oral polio vaccine (OPV)** with virus grown in tissue culture (e.g., monkey kidney or human diploid cells). This vaccine provides more complete protection by developing both intestinal and humoral immunity.

    (5) Rabies vaccine is currently available in two forms.

        (a) Virus grown in duck embryo is inactivated with β-propiolactone for use as a vaccine. This vaccine is not always free of neurologic complications.

        (b) Virus grown in nerve tissue-free human diploid cells (i.e., human lung fibroblasts) is inactivated with tributyl phosphate and is the preferred vaccine.

    (6) Hepatitis B vaccine is composed of inactivated, alum-adsorbed hepatitis B surface antigen (HB_sAg) particles purified from plasma of human carriers. HB_sAg produced by a genetically engineered strain of *Saccharomyces cerevisiae* is also available as vaccine.

  b. Rickettsial

    (1) Typhus vaccine is prepared from formalin-killed *Rickettsia prowazekii* grown in the yolk sac of chick embryos.

    (2) Rocky Mountain spotted fever vaccine is prepared from formalin-killed *Rickettsia rickettsii* grown in chick embryos.

IV. PASSIVE IMMUNIZATION (IMMUNOTHERAPY).
Passive, artificially acquired immunity is effective and acts immediately, but is only temporary in its effect. Three basic types of serum preparations are used—antitoxin, immune globulin, and specific immune globulin.

  A. Antitoxins consist of toxin-neutralizing antibodies (antiserum) specific for a given toxin. They have no effect on the microorganism that produced the toxin.

    1. Most commercial preparations are produced by immunizing (with toxin or toxoid) horses or cows, harvesting the serum or plasma, and processing it to concentrate the antitoxin and eliminate as much horse or cow serum protein as possible. The preparations are then sterilized by filtration, treated with a chemical preservative, and standardized.

    2. Representative currently used preparations

      a. Botulism is treated by the administration of polyvalent antitoxin to three types (types A, B, and E) of toxin produced by *Clostridium botulinum*. The antitoxin is prepared in horses.

      b. Diphtheria antitoxin (DAT) is prepared in horses by injection of toxoid of *C. diphtheriae*, and is effective in the treatment of cases of diphtheria. (For prevention of diphtheria, see section III A 3 a.)

      c. Tetanus is treated by human-derived specific immune globulin that is specific for the toxin of *C. tetani*. Animal-derived antitoxins are available but not recommended.

  B. Immune globulin (IG), also referred to as **gamma globulin**, is prepared from pooled normal adult human plasma or serum by cold ethanol fractionation. It contains a variety of different antibodies (mainly IgG) to several microorganisms and is used for passive immunization against those diseases or for maintenance of immunodeficient individuals. Hepatitis A (infectious hepatitis or short incubation hepatitis) and measles immune globulins are both human-derived.

  C. Specific immune globulin (SIG) is a gamma globulin obtained from individuals who have recently recovered from a specific infectious disease or from hyperimmunized human volunteers.

    1. Hepatitis B immune globulin (HBIG) is derived from human plasma that demonstrates a high titer of antibody to HB_sAg.

    2. Rabies immune globulin (RIG) is serum prepared from humans who have been hyperimmunized against rabies (usually veterinarians), for use in treating individuals exposed to rabid animals. Rabies immune globulin is used in conjunction with rabies vaccine.

    3. Varicella-zoster immune globulin (VZIG), prepared from human-derived serum selected for high titers of antibody to varicella-zoster, will modify or prevent varicella (chickenpox) in immunodeficient children but is of no benefit to persons with active varicella or herpes zoster (shingles).

    4. Rh immune globulin is a human-derived preparation used in Rh-negative women within 72 hours of delivery, miscarriage, or abortion of an Rh-positive baby or fetus to prevent sensitization of the mother to possible Rh-positive fetal red blood cells in future pregnancies.

V. EXPERIMENTAL IMMUNIZATION PROCEDURES.
Concern over currently used immunization techniques, particularly their safety and efficacy, has resulted in the development of various

means to augment the immune response (immunopotentiation) either specifically or nonspecifically and in the development of a number of newer vaccines. Some examples are presented here.

A. Nonspecific immunopotentiation

1. **Bacille Calmette-Guérin (BCG)** is a live attenuated strain of *M. bovis* used with varying degrees of success to immunize against tuberculosis. Through its ability to nonspecifically stimulate the immune response, administration of BCG can also inhibit the development or induce regression of certain malignant tumors. It can be given by intradermal injection or by the scarification method, either alone or in conjunction with chemotherapy.
   a. BCG appears to activate T cells and macrophages and stimulate **natural killer (NK) cells**. Further, it cross-reacts antigenically with certain tumor cells, suggesting the possibility that it might also stimulate a specific antitumor immune response.
   b. In certain types of cancer (e.g., malignant melanoma, acute lymphocytic leukemia, acute myelogenous leukemia), BCG administration has resulted in some arrest of spread and some prolongation of disease-free intervals.
   c. The sometimes severe side effects of its use [e.g., chills, fever, anaphylaxis, and occasional BCG infection (in immunosuppressed individuals)] have led to attempts to prepare purified subfractions of the organism designed to reduce such complications. A methanol-extractable residue of phenol-treated BCG (MER–BCG) appears to have some promise. Muramyl dipeptide (MDP), a cell wall fraction, is also under investigation.

2. *Corynebacterium parvum*, a gram-positive bacterium, is used as a heat-killed, formaldehyde-treated suspension. Given orally or injected parenterally (intralesionally), it is reported to cause regression of certain tumors (e.g., malignant melanoma), probably by activating macrophages. Undesirable side effects include fever and vomiting.

3. **Levamisole** is a potent anthelmintic drug that is also an interesting immunostimulant. It appears to augment depressed T-cell mediated immunity and enhance phagocytosis. Clinical studies have shown levamisole to be of limited value in such conditions as herpesvirus infection, staphylococcal infections, and certain types of cancer. Complications include nausea, rash, and neutropenia.

4. **Interferon** was originally associated with antiviral effects; however, it is now recognized as having important immunoregulatory properties. Three classes of interferon—alpha, beta, and gamma—have been identified. Its major immunoregulatory effect seems to be enhancement of NK cells and macrophages. It is species-specific and, hence, human-derived material must be used in humans. Recently, production of interferon in *Escherichia coli* by recombinant DNA technology has been reported. Interferon has been found to be of some value in osteosarcoma and other types of tumors, herpesvirus infection, hepatitis, and the common cold. Occasional leukopenia and fever may complicate its use.

5. **Interleukin-2** is a mitogenic lymphokine produced by T cells that stimulates growth of activated T cells and converts quiescent cells into active cytotoxic cells that are referred to as **lymphokine activated killer (LAK) cells**. Interleukin-2 also appears to augment NK-cell cytotoxicity, possibly via stimulation of interferon production. Clinical trials of its effectiveness in the management of certain types of cancer are in progress.

B. Specific immunization. Numerous attempts to develop both new and improved vaccines, as well as techniques for antigen-specific immune modulation, are currently in progress.

1. **Pneumococcal pneumonia.** Mutants of *S. pneumoniae* able to colonize the upper respiratory tract are under investigation, as are attempts to improve immunogenicity of the polysaccharide capsule by coupling it to protein.

2. **Group A streptococci and their products** are associated with sore throat, endocarditis, rheumatic fever, glomerulonephritis, and other diseases. **Type-specific M protein** (an antiphagocytic virulence factor), freed of toxic and tissue cross-reactive materials by salt fractionation and ion-exchange chromatography, is being evaluated as a vaccine.

3. **Group B streptococci**, particularly serotype III, are a major cause of neonatal meningitis. Purified capsular polysaccharide prepared from type III organisms has been found to be well tolerated and immunogenic, and is being investigated as an immunizing agent for the mother to provide protective antibody levels to the newborn.

4. **Gonococcal infection.** Despite exhaustive control efforts by public and private health facilities, rates of infection caused by *N. gonorrhoeae* remain high and emphasize the need for a vaccine. Attachment of gonococci to host tissue is an important part of the disease process. Only types 1 and 2 appear to be virulent and possess pili that facilitate attachment. Antibody against pili not only blocks attachment but also enhances phagocytosis of gonococci. It is pos-

sible that pili can be used as an immunogen to protect against gonococcal infection. The existence of multiple antigenic types of pili may pose a problem.

5. **Meningococcal meningitis.** Immunity to infection by *Neisseria meningitidis* is associated with complement-dependent bactericidal antibodies. The antibodies are group-specific.
   a. The protection-inducing antigen for groups A and C meningococci is capsular polysaccharide. Group A and group C polysaccharides are relatively poor immunogens in young infants.
   b. The protection-inducing antigen for group B appears to be a type-specific protein. Group B polysaccharide is poorly immunogenic.
   c. Studies aimed at enhancing the immunogenicity of capsular material by coupling it to protein (e.g., tetanus toxoid) are in progress.

6. **Typhoid fever.** The current vaccine for typhoid fever, whole killed *S. typhi*, affords only partial resistance and is considerably toxic. Oral administration of a live attenuated mutant strain has been studied in controlled field trials and found to be extremely effective.

7. **Enterotoxigenic *E. coli* (ETEC)** appears to be a major cause of traveler's diarrhea, or "turista," precipitated by an enterotoxin-induced hypersecretion in the small intestine. The plasmids carrying genes for enterotoxins may also carry genes for colonization factors that aid attachment of organisms to intestinal epithelium. Both toxin and colonization factor antigens (CFA) are being examined for use as vaccine.

8. ***H. influenzae* disease (bacterial meningitis).** Unfortunately, the currently used vaccine (polysaccharide capsule of *H. influenzae* type b) is not effective in infants younger than age 18 months, the age-group that suffers the highest attack rate. The immunogenicity of the capsular material can be increased by conjugating it to a protein carrier. Tetanus toxoid as a carrier is under investigation.

9. **Cholera.** The limited protection against cholera conferred by conventional vaccine (killed *Vibrio cholerae*) has led to the development of experimental vaccines. New approaches include combined antigens consisting of toxoid or a subunit of toxin together with conventional vaccine or *Vibrio* lipopolysaccharide. Avirulent mutants of *V. cholerae* are also under investigation for use as live oral vaccine.

10. ***Pseudomonas aeruginosa*** is an important pathogen that can cause serious wound and burn infections, meningitis, urinary tract infection, ear infection, and others. Detoxified lipopolysaccharide, lipopolysaccharide–protein conjugates, and toxoid are being evaluated as vaccines.

11. **Anti-idiotypic antibody vaccines.** Immunoglobulin idiotypes represent unique amino acid sequences in the variable region associated with the antigen-binding capability of the molecule. Idiotypic sites are capable of inducing antibody production (i.e., anti-idiotypic antibody). In recent years, it has been found that anti-idiotypic antibodies directed at the variable region, specifically the hypervariable site, of antimicrobial antibodies can be used as vaccines since the anti-idiotypic preparation contains an internal image component that mimics the epitope of the microbial antigen. Anti-idiotypic antibodies have been used to induce an immune response in experimental animals in a variety of systems (e.g., trypanosomiasis, rabies, reovirus, Sendai virus, polio, herpes, and hepatitis B).

12. **Immunotoxins**, which are produced by linking toxins to highly specific monoclonal antibodies, have shown promise in recent experimental studies. A popular toxin used is ricin, extracted from castor bean plants, which can inhibit protein synthesis and cause cell death. An immunotoxin that could be of potential value in cancer therapy would be one consisting of ricin coupled to monoclonal antibody specific for tumor cell antigens. Such a preparation should have no effect on normal tissue. Another area of investigation is the management of autoimmune disease. In the disease myasthenia gravis, neuromuscular transmission is impaired because the patient makes antiacetylcholine receptor antibodies. The goal of studies in progress is to construct an immunotoxin that would eliminate the set of lymphocytes that make antiacetylcholine receptor antibody.

13. **Transfer factor (TF)** is a dialyzable, low molecular weight nucleopeptide derived from activated T cells, which is capable of transferring antigen-specific, cell-mediated immunity and delayed skin test reactivity from specifically sensitized donors to nonsensitized recipients. To date, TF has been reported to be of some clinical value in the management of certain viral diseases (e.g., measles, herpes, and chickenpox in childhood leukemia), fungal infections (e.g., mucocutaneous candidiasis and histoplasmosis), bacterial diseases (e.g., tuberculosis), parasitic infections (e.g., leishmaniasis), and cancers (e.g., osteosarcoma and malignant melanoma).

STUDY QUESTIONS

Directions: Each question below contains five suggested answers. Choose the **one best** response to each question.

1. The preferred vaccine for diphtheria consists of

(A) heat-killed *Corynebacterium diphtheriae*
(B) precipitated adsorbed toxoid
(C) attenuated *C. diphtheriae*
(D) capsular polysaccharide
(E) capsule plus carrier protein

2. Bacille Calmette-Guérin (BCG) is sometimes used for

(A) passive immunization for tuberculosis
(B) inducing production of neutralizing antibody
(C) nonspecific suppression of the immune response
(D) inducing antipili antibody production
(E) nonspecific protentiation of the immune response

3. The major immunoregulatory effect of interferon seems to be

(A) differentiation of plasma cells
(B) enhancement of natural killer (NK) cells and macrophages
(C) suppression of cell-mediated immunity
(D) enhancement of antibody production
(E) provision of passive immunity

4. An immune response that mimics the response induced by natural infection is believed to be stimulated by administering agents via the

(A) subcutaneous route
(B) percutaneous route
(C) intradermal route
(D) intramuscular route
(E) intranasal route

Directions: Each question below contains four suggested answers of which **one or more** is correct. Choose the answer

A   if **1, 2, and 3** are correct
B   if **1 and 3** are correct
C   if **2 and 4** are correct
D   if **4** is correct
E   if **1, 2, 3, and 4** are correct

5. Purified polysaccharide capsule is used to vaccinate against infection caused by

(1) *Bordetella pertussis*
(2) *Haemophilus influenzae*
(3) *Salmonella typhi*
(4) *Streptococcus pneumoniae*

6. Active artificial immunization (immunoprophylaxis) is induced by the administration of

(1) bacterial products
(2) toxoids
(3) vaccines
(4) antitoxins

7. Specific immune globulin (SIG) is preferred for passive immunization against

(1) tetanus
(2) rabies
(3) chickenpox (varicella)
(4) botulism

8. Agents used for nonspecific immunopotentiation include

(1) interleukin-2
(2) anti-idiotypic antibody
(3) *Corynebacterium parvum*
(4) immunotoxins

9. Live attenuated virus composes the vaccine used for

(1) rubella
(2) measles
(3) poliomyelitis
(4) serum hepatitis

10. Transfer factor (TF) is a nucleopeptide that is

(1) derived from activated T cells
(2) involved in passive cutaneous anaphylaxis
(3) capable of transferring cell-mediated immunity
(4) involved in the Prausnitz-Küstner reaction

Directions: The group of questions below consists of lettered choices followed by several numbered items. For each numbered item select the **one** lettered choice with which it is **most** closely associated. Each lettered choice may be used once, more than once, or not at all.

Questions 11–14

Match each description of an immunizing agent to the type of vaccine it best characterizes.

(A) Bacterial vaccines
(B) Rickettsial vaccines
(C) Antitoxins
(D) Immune globulin (IG)
(E) Specific immune globulin (SIG)

11. Contain products that are detoxified

12. Contain natural fluid plain toxoid

13. Prepared from hyperimmunized human volunteers

14. Prepared from pooled normal adult human plasma

ANSWERS AND EXPLANATIONS

1. The answer is B. (*III A 3 a*) The preferred vaccine for diphtheria is fluid toxoid precipitated with potassium alum or adsorbed onto aluminum hydroxide or phosphate. Since diphtheria results primarily from the action of the toxin formed by *Corynebacterium diphtheriae* rather than from invasion by the organism, resistance to the disease depends on specific neutralizing antitoxin such as that induced by vaccination.

2. The answer is E. (*V A 1*) Bacille Calmette-Guerin (BCG) is a live attenuated strain of *Mycobacterium bovis* used with varying degrees of success to actively immunize against tuberculosis. Administration of BCG can also nonspecifically stimulate the immune response. It appears to activate T cells and macrophages and to stimulate natural killer (NK) cells. Its primary effect is on cell-mediated immunity, not humoral antibody-mediated immunity.

3. The answer is B. (*V A 4*) Interferon, while it was originally associated with antiviral effects, is now recognized as having important immunoregulatory properties, mainly enhancement of natural killer (NK) cells and macrophages. It would thus be expected to enhance cell-mediated immunity but have little effect on humoral antibody-mediated immunity.

4. The answer is E. (*II C*) Recent applications of immunization via intranasal administration indicate that, particularly in upper respiratory disease, an immune response can be stimulated that mimics a response induced by a natural infection; that is, one resulting in the production of specific antibodies both in serum and secretions at the local site of infection. Evaluation of the intranasal route of administration for influenza vaccination is currently underway.

5. The answer is C (2, 4). (*III A 3 b, e–g*) Polysaccharide capsular material is used to vaccinate against pneumococcal pneumonia and against bacterial meningitis caused by *Haemophilus influenzae* type b. Vaccines for typhoid fever (*Salmonella typhi*) and pertussis (*Bordetella pertussis*) consist of intact killed organisms.

6. The answer is A (1, 2, 3). (*III A 1, 2*) Active artificially acquired immunity is induced by the use of vaccines which consist of either intact microorganisms (killed or attenuated) or their component parts (e.g., capsule) or products (e.g., toxoid) which are unable to produce disease but are still antigenic and able to induce an immune response. Antitoxins are used to induce passive, not active, immunity.

7. The answer is A (1, 2, 3). (*IV A 2 a, c, C 2, 3*) Specific immune globulin (SIG), which is gamma globulin obtained from persons who have recently recovered from a specific infectious disease or from hyperimmunized human volunteers, is used for passive immunization against tetanus, rabies, and chickenpox (varicella). In the case of botulism, antitoxin prepared in horses is used.

8. The answer is B (1, 3). (*V A 2, 5, B 11, 12*) Interleukin-2 and *Corynebacterium parvum* both nonspecifically stimulate the immune response, the former by inducing production of lymphokine activated killer (LAK) cells and augmenting natural killer (NK)-cell activity and the latter by activating macrophages. Anti-idiotypic antibody and immunotoxins are used for antigen-specific suppression of the immune response.

9. The answer is A (1, 2, 3). [*III B 3 a (1), (3), (4), (6)*] Live attenuated virus grown in tissue culture or chick embryo is used to vaccinate against rubella (German measles), measles (rubeola), and polio (Sabin vaccine). An inactivated virus preparation (Salk vaccine) is also available for polio. Serum hepatitis (hepatitis B) vaccine consists of chemically inactivated, adsorbed surface antigen particles purified from plasma of human carriers. Surface antigen produced by genetically engineered *Saccharomyces cerevisiae* is also available.

10. The answer is B (1, 3). (*V B 13*) Transfer factor (TF) is a dialyzable, low molecular weight nucleopeptide derived from activated T cells, which is capable of transferring antigen-specific, cell-mediated immunity and delayed skin test reactivity from specifically sensitized donors to nonsensitized recipients. Passive cutaneous anaphylaxis and the Prausnitz-Kustner reaction are passive transfer tests used to assay cytotropic antibody.

11–14. The answers are: 11-A, 12-A, 13-E, 14-D. (*III A 2 b; IV C, B*) Bacterial products used for immunization are usually structural components or detoxified products known as toxoids.

Toxoids are toxins that are converted (via heat or formaldehyde treatment) into nontoxic but immunogenic materials that are called natural fluid plain toxoid, which induces the production of antitoxic antibodies.

   Specific immune globulin (SIG) is a gamma globulin otained from persons who have recently recovered from a specific infectious disease or from human volunteers who have been hyperimmunized.
   Immune globulin (IG), or gamma globulin, is prepared from pooled normal adult human plasma or serum by cold ethanol fractionation. IG is used for passive immunization or for maintenance of immunodeficient persons, and contains antibodies to the most common infectious agents that affect humans (e.g., measles and rubella).

8
Laboratory Methods

I. INTRODUCTION. In vitro **antigen–antibody reactions** (i.e., serologic reactions) provide methods for the diagnosis of disease and for the identification and quantitation of antigens and antibodies.

    A. The titer, or level, of antibody in serum can be measured by using known antigens, and such titers can be of diagnostic and prognostic importance (e.g., a rise in antibody titer between acute and convalescent serum can be diagnostic for a specific disease).

    B. The forces involved in antigen–antibody interactions are profoundly affected by various environmental factors.

        1. Physiologic pH and salt concentration promote optimal union. Forces of attraction tend to be weaker in acid (below pH 4.0) and alkaline (above pH 10.0) conditions.

        2. Temperature also plays an important role: the higher the temperature (up to a maximum of 50–55°C), the more rapid the rate of reaction. This is due to the increase in kinetic motion of the reactants.

    C. The physical state of the antigen is responsible, in general, for the identification of antigen–antibody reactions and the naming of antibodies.

        1. Agglutinins are antibodies that aggregate cellular antigens.

        2. Lysins are antibodies that cause dissolution of cell membranes.

        3. Precipitins are antibodies that form precipitates with soluble antigens.

        4. Antitoxins are antibodies that neutralize toxins.

II. PROCEDURES INVOLVING DIRECT DEMONSTRATION AND OBSERVATION OF REACTIONS. The relative sensitivities of the tests for antigens and antibodies are presented in Table 8-1.

Table 8-1. Relative Sensitivity of Tests Measuring Antibody and Antigen

Test	Approximate Detectable Amount (μg/ml)	
	Antibody	Antigen
Precipitation	20.0	1.0
Immunoelectrophoresis	20.0	. . .
Double diffusion in agar gel	1.0	. . .
Complement fixation	0.5	. . .
Radial immunodiffusion	0.05	0.5
Bacterial agglutination	0.01	. . .
Hemolysis	0.01	. . .
Passive hemagglutination	0.01	. . .
Hemagglutination inhibition	. . .	0.001
Antitoxin neutralization	0.01	. . .
Radioimmunoassay	0.0005	0.000005
Enzyme-linked immunosorbent assay	0.0005	0.000005
Virus neutralization	0.00005	. . .

A. Agglutination. Agglutination reactions serve to detect and quantitate **agglutinins** and identify **cellular** antigens. Agglutinins are antibodies that agglutinate cellular structures, including bacterial cells, white blood cells, and red blood cells. When the cells interact with the appropriate antibody, they clump together and eventually form masses that become large enough to be seen. When antibody agglutinates bacteria in the body, **opsonization** occurs.

1. Agglutination occurs because antibodies are at least **bivalent** (i.e., they have at least two combining sites).

2. Two sites on the antibody and multiple sites on the antigen result in **antigen–antibody lattice** formation that can build up into increasingly larger complexes (Fig. 8-1). The aggregates may be seen in the test tube or under the microscope.

3. A classic example of the application of the agglutination reaction is seen in the **Widal test** in the diagnosis of typhoid fever.
    a. In this test, the antibody content of the patient's serum is measured by adding a constant amount of antigen (e.g., *Salmonella typhi*) to serially diluted serum.
    b. After appropriate incubation, the tubes are examined for visible agglutination. The last tube (i.e., highest dilution of serum) showing agglutination is referred to as the **titer**.

B. Lysis. In the presence of complement, an antigen–antibody reaction on a cell membrane may result in membrane damage leading to **cell lysis**, presumed to be due to the enzymatic activity of the activated complement. The phenomenon is probably of importance in the host's defense against microbial infections, cancer, and so forth.

1. **Hemolysis**, in which the hemoglobin is released from the red blood cell, is a requisite phenomenon for the **complement fixation test**.

2. Cells of gram-negative bacteria also undergo immune lysis, referred to as **bacteriolysis**, under certain conditions.

3. **Cytolysis** involves the destruction of other cell types (e.g., tumor cells) under appropriate conditions in the presence of specific antibody and complement.

C. Precipitation occurs when the antigen is **soluble** instead of cellular. Therefore, a large number of molecules are required for lattice formation, and a large lattice must be formed in order for an aggregate to be visible.

1. When soluble antigens come in contact with specific antibody, they aggregate (precipitate) (Fig. 8-2).
    a. Where the antigen concentration is very low with a relative superabundance of antibody (**zone of antibody excess**), formation of complexes occurs, but residual antibody will remain in the **supernatant**. This area is known as a **prozone**.
    b. As more antigen is added, large aggregates form. In the **zone of equivalence**, there is neither antigen nor antibody in the supernatant.
    c. Instead of reaching a plateau, this curve comes back down to zero with increasing amounts of antigen (**zone of antigen excess**) because the lattice size becomes too small to precipitate.

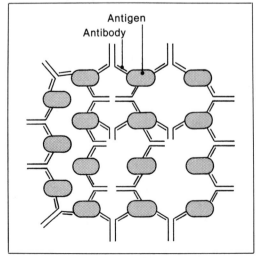

Figure 8-1. Lattice structure composed of antigen and antibody.

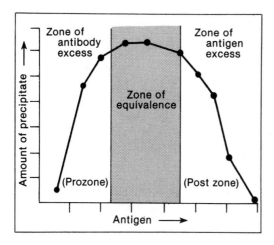

Figure 8-2. Effect of increasing amounts of antigen on total immune precipitate obtained in mixture of soluble antigen and its homologous antibody.

    (1) In extreme antigen excess, the complex will be **trimolecular** (i.e., one antibody and two antigens). When soluble complexes form in vivo, they may cause a disease called **serum sickness**.
        (a) An example of this is the administration of diphtheria antitoxin made from horse serum, which is a foreign protein to humans.
        (b) People given too much antitoxin (i.e., antigen) may develop serum sickness.
    (2) The soluble complexes are not handled well by the **reticuloendothelial system**.

2. Precipitation can also be demonstrated via **immunodiffusion**. If an antigen–antibody reaction takes place in a semisolid medium (e.g., agar), bands of precipitate will form because of the diffusion of the components toward each other. A useful example of this is a **double immunodiffusion method** called the **Ouchterlony technique**.
    a. Antigen and antibody preparations are placed in separate wells that are cut into a thin layer of agar in a petri dish.
    b. The reactants diffuse toward each other through the agar until they meet at optimal proportions and form **bands of precipitate** (Fig. 8-3).
    c. The advantage of the procedure is that **antigenic relationships can be detected by the precipitation pattern**. The three basic patterns are illustrated in Figure 8-4.
        (1) In **reactions of identity**, if the two antigens are identical, they will diffuse at the same rate, and the two precipitin bands merge into a solid chevron.
        (2) In **reactions of nonidentity**, the two antigens are completely different, and the lines of precipitate cross.
        (3) The **reaction of partial identity** is indicated by **spur formation**, indicating that one of the antigens is cross-reactive with, but not identical to, the other. The spur occurs because one of the antibodies does not react with the cross-reacting antigen but migrates past that antigen until it reaches an antigen with the epitope for which it has specificity. The spur in Figure 8-4 contains antibody **b** only; antibody **a** reacted with epitope a on antigen ac.

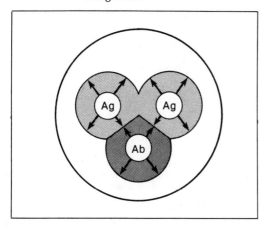

Figure 8-3. Diffusion of reactants in two-dimensional immunodiffusion. *Ag* = antigen; *Ab* = antibody.

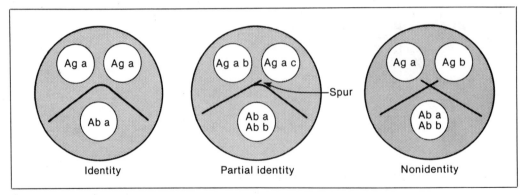

Figure 8-4. Types of patterns seen in immunodiffusion. *Ag* = antigen; *Ab* = antibody.

3. **Quantitative radial immunodiffusion** is a variation of the immunodiffusion phenomenon that provides for quantitation of antigens. It is used routinely to quantitate human serum immunoglobulins.
   a. For this purpose, an agar-coated slide is used, the agar being impregnated by antiserum (e.g., antibody to human IgG). Serum samples are then placed in wells in the agar.
   b. As it diffuses through the agar and encounters the antibody, the IgG in the sample will form a concentric ring, or **halo of precipitate**. The diameter of the halo of precipitate directly correlates with the concentration of IgG in the sample. The level of IgG in the sample can be determined by reference to a standard curve based on halo diameters of known concentrations of IgG.

4. The double-diffusion technique could not always resolve highly complex mixtures of antigens; therefore, a more sophisticated technique was developed, called **immunoelectrophoresis**.
   a. In this procedure, antigen is placed in wells in agar on a glass slide and then subjected to electrophoresis via application of an electric current.
   b. Under these conditions, the individual antigenic components will migrate through the agar at variable rates. If antibody is then placed in a well running the length of the slide and parallel to the path of migration, the reactants will diffuse toward one another and form **separate arcs of precipitate** for each antigenic component.

5. **Counterimmunoelectrophoresis** is another variant procedure. This technique is the double-diffusion method with the addition of an electric current as the migratory force, which greatly amplifies the speed of the reaction (30–90 minutes) and intensifies the precipitin bands.
   a. Antigen and antibody are placed in wells and current is applied.
   b. In suitable buffer, the negatively charged antigen migrates toward the anode, whereas the antibody (with no significant net charge) migrates in the opposite, or counter, direction as a result of **endosmosis**. Precipitation occurs where the reactants meet.

D. **Toxin–antitoxin reactions.** If a serum contains an **antitoxin** (i.e., an antibody to a toxin), the antibody will neutralize the toxin.

1. The presence of antibody to diphtheria toxin can be easily measured using the **Schick test**, which is used to test for immunity to diphtheria.
   a. The presence or absence of antitoxin in an individual's serum can be shown by injecting intradermally a small amount of the toxin. If there is antibody, there should be no reaction.
   b. A **positive** test indicates the absence of antibody; a **negative** test indicates that there was sufficient antitoxin to neutralize the toxin injected.

2. Antitoxin can also be detected via **neutralization in vitro**. If, for example, serum containing antitoxin is mixed with toxin in vitro, and then, after a few minutes, a small amount of the mixture is injected into an experimental animal, the animal will be protected against the deleterious effects of the toxin.

E. **Flocculation** is another form of antigen–antibody reaction that occurs if the antigen is neither cellular nor soluble, but is an insoluble particulate. The **Venereal Disease Research Laboratory (VDRL) test** is a slide flocculation test used for the diagnosis of syphilis.

1. The VDRL test makes use of a **heterogenetic (heterophil) antigen** shared between the spirochete of syphilis and normal beef heart. The antigen used is a **water-insoluble cardio-**

lipin that has coated the surface of cholesterol particles added to the system. These form visible aggregates in the presence of an antibody (**reagin**) in the serum of patients with syphilis.

2. The test may be performed on a glass slide or on commercially available cards via the **rapid plasma reagin (RPR) test**.

III. COMPLEX SEROLOGIC PROCEDURES. Antigen–antibody reactions in which the visible manifestation requires the participation of accessory factors, indicator systems, and specialized equipment can be measured by several techniques.

A. **Complement fixation. Complement**, a protein constituent of normal blood serum, is consumed (fixed) during the interaction of antigens and antibodies. This phenomenon forms the basis for the **complement fixation test**, a sensitive test that can be used to detect and quantitate antigens and antibodies.

1. The primary reacting ingredients are antigen, antibody, and complement.
   a. **Normal guinea pig serum** is often used as a primary source of complement due to the animal's high levels of complement having efficient lytic properties.
   b. Different sources of complement are used in differing in vitro tests (e.g., rabbit complement is used in cytotoxicity tests performed for transplantation).

2. To use the complement fixation test to determine the presence of antibody to a given, known antigen in a patient's serum, a test system and indicator system are used.
   a. **Test system.** To the serum (heated to 56°C to inactivate native complement) is added measured amounts of antigen and complement (guinea pig serum). If antibody specific for the known antigen is present in the serum, antigen–antibody complexes will be formed that will fix all the complement. The initial reaction, however, cannot be seen.
   b. **Indicator system.** In a second step, an indicator system consisting of sheep red blood cells (SRBCs) plus **hemolysin**, an antibody specific for SRBCs, is added to test for the presence of free complement. Interpretation of the test is based on the presence of hemolysis.
      (1) If all the complement has been fixed, none will be free to lyse the SRBCs, which constitutes a **positive complement fixation test**.
      (2) If no antibody is present in the patient's serum, then the complement is not fixed and is free to interact in the indicator system and lyse the SRBCs, which constitutes a **negative complement fixation test**.

3. Properly conducted complement fixation tests require the incorporation of appropriate **controls** to assure that the results will not be adversely affected by the presence of **anticomplementary ingredients**. The antigen or the serum itself may have anticomplementary properties (e.g., denatured or aggregated immunoglobulin, heparin, chelating agents, or microbial contaminants); may fix all the complement in the system; or may remove calcium or magnesium ions, both of which are essential for complement-mediated lysis.

B. **Immunofluorescence.** Fluorescent dyes (e.g., fluorescein isothiocyanate) can be conjugated to antibody molecules to allow visualization of the molecules **via ultraviolet light and a fluorescence microscope**. Such **labeled antibody** may then be used to identify antigens. Both direct and indirect techniques are available.

1. **Direct immunofluorescence** employs antibody specific for a particular antigen or parasite labeled with a fluorescent dye, usually fluorescein. This is allowed to react with an unknown tissue or organism. If the antibody reacts, it will be visualized as a green stain on the specimen when it is examined under ultraviolet light. For the identification of *Treponema pallidum* in an exudate from a patient suspected of having syphilis, the following procedure would be used.
   a. A slide of exudate is prepared and flooded with tagged, specific antibody. If organisms are present in the exudate, they will bind the tagged antibody.
   b. Excess antibody is then washed from the slide, and the slide is examined with a fluorescence microscope; *T. pallidum* will fluoresce against the black background. This is a remarkably rapid, useful test for the identification of unknown microorganisms.

2. **Indirect immunofluorescence** procedures employ antibody against antibody (e.g., rabbit antihuman gamma globulin antiserum) which has a fluorescent compound covalently coupled to it.
   a. The "**sandwich technique**" allows for **detection of antibody**.
      (1) In the serodiagnosis of syphilis by the **fluorescent treponemal antibody absorption (FTA-ABS) test**, *T. pallidum* fixed to a slide is flooded with patient's serum to be tested for antibody. If antibodies to the spirochete are present, they will bind to the organisms on the slide.

    (2) Excess antibody is removed by washing, and to detect bound antibody, the preparation is overlaid with fluorescein-tagged antibody to human gamma globulin. If the patient's serum contains antibody to *T. pallidum*, fluorescing organisms will be seen when the slide is examined with the fluorescence microscope.

    b. Indirect immunofluorescence is also used in detecting **antinuclear antibodies** (e.g., DNA, RNA, and histone). Antinuclear antibodies are present in systemic lupus erythematosus (SLE), and sometimes in rheumatoid arthritis and other autoimmune collagen–vascular diseases. For diagnosing SLE, the procedure is essentially identical to that described above for *T. pallidum* except that the antigen is DNA in forms such as animal or human buffy coat cells, rat kidney sections, and beef thymus sections.

C. Hemagglutination inhibition. Hemagglutination involves the agglutination of red blood cells by antibodies (i.e., **hemagglutinins**), certain virus particles (e.g., influenza and mumps viruses), or other substances. Although viral hemagglutination is a nonimmunologic phenomenon, it forms the basis for the **hemagglutination inhibition test**, an extremely valuable viral diagnostic test.

    1. The test is valuable for demonstrating the presence of serum antibody to hemagglutinating viral substances. Similar tests can be employed to detect soluble antigens that react with and neutralize a hemagglutinating antibody (see section III D 4).

    2. To examine the serum of a patient suspected of having influenza for influenza antibody, the patient's serum is mixed with known influenza virus and red blood cells.
        a. If antibody is present, hemagglutination will be inhibited due to the ability of the antibody to bind to the virus and block its ability to hemagglutinate:

$$\text{Serum antibody + Virus + Red blood cells} \rightarrow \text{No hemagglutination.}$$

        b. If no antibody is present, hemagglutination will occur:

$$\text{Virus + Red blood cells} \rightarrow \text{Hemagglutination.}$$

D. Passive agglutination is the conversion of a reaction system from one that precipitates to one that agglutinates, thus yielding a more sensitive indication of antibody.

    1. The use of **latex particles** in the diagnosis of **rheumatoid arthritis** is an example of passive agglutination. In this disease, the patient produces an antibody (mainly IgM) to his own IgG. The test consists of coating latex particles with IgG and reacting them with the patient's serum. Agglutination indicates the presence of antibodies, or a **positive test**.

    2. Bis-diazotized benzidine is a coupling reagent that can be used to conjugate proteins or haptens to red blood cells, thus allowing the detection of specific antibodies to these materials by passive hemagglutination procedures.

    3. In the **Rose-Waaler test** for the detection of **rheumatoid factor** in serum (an anti-IgG autoantibody), tannic acid-treated SRBCs are coated with rabbit IgG antibodies specific for the SRBCs.

    4. Antibodies to a soluble antigen such as IgG will cause the agglutination of red blood cells that have IgG coupled to their membranes. However, if soluble IgG is added to the antiserum before the IgG-coated red blood cells are admixed, the anti-IgG antibody will react with the soluble antigen and hemagglutination will be inhibited.

E. Coombs (antiglobulin) test. In certain cases, antibodies directed against antigenic determinants are unable to form visible aggregates when subjected to precipitation or agglutination procedures. In order to demonstrate the presence of antibody in such cases, the Coombs (antiglobulin) test may be employed. The Coombs test involves adding an antibody directed against gamma globulin, thus providing a bridge between two antibody-coated cells or particles. The test is performed in two ways.

    1. The **direct Coombs test** is used to detect cell-bound antibody. The red blood cells are washed free of serum and unbound antibody, and the antiglobulin reagent is added directly to the cell suspension. The direct Coombs test is of value in the detection of antibodies to red blood cells associated with syndromes such as **hemolytic disease of the newborn (erythroblastosis fetalis)** and **autoimmune hemolytic disease**. The antibodies associated with these diseases have the ability to attach to, but not agglutinate, the target red blood cell. The absorbed antibody (gamma globulin) can be detected, however, by the use of an antibody (**Coombs serum**) to human gamma globulin.

    2. The **indirect Coombs test** is used to detect the presence of circulating nonagglutinating antibody. A serum sample is incubated with donor red blood cells, the cells are washed, and the antiglobulin reagent is added. If antibody has adsorbed to the red blood cells, they will now be agglutinated. The indirect Coombs test is of value in detecting IgG-associated antibody in the serum of a woman who is thought to be sensitized to the Rh antigen and at risk for carrying an erythroblastotic fetus.

F. Viral neutralization is very similar to hemagglutination inhibition, and in fact the latter is a "neutralization" event. The assays are based on the ability of specific antibodies to interfere with some biological function of the virus. Usually the viral property blocked is **infectivity**.

1. Certain viruses (e.g., herpes virus), when added to appropriate target cells growing in tissue culture (e.g., rabbit kidney cells), will produce observable cell destruction referred to as **cytopathic effects (CPE)**.

2. The phenomenon of CPE is useful in the search for **virus-neutralizing antibodies** in a serum sample. The serum suspected of containing antibody is added to a virus suspension and then a susceptible cell culture is inoculated with the mixture.
   a. If the cell culture fails to develop a CPE, then antibodies were present in the serum sample:

   Serum antibody + Virus + Target cell → No CPE.

   b. If CPE develops, then no neutralizing antibodies were present:

   Virus + Target cell → CPE.

G. Radioimmunoassay (RIA) is an extremely sensitive method that can be used for the quantitation of any substance that is **immunogenic or haptenic** and can be **labeled with a radioactive isotope** [e.g., iodine 125 (^{125}I)]. The method is capable of measuring picogram quantities or less, depending on the substance being assayed.

1. **Liquid-phase RIA** depends on the competition between **labeled (known)** and **unlabeled (unknown) antigen** for the same antibody.
   a. A known amount of labeled antigen, a known amount of specific antibody, and an unknown amount of unlabeled antigen are allowed to react together. The antigen–antibody complexes that form are then separated out by either physicochemical or immunologic means (e.g., ammonium sulfate or second antibody precipitation, respectively), and their radioactivity is determined.
   b. By measuring the radioactivity still remaining in the supernatant (unbound, labeled antigen), the percentage of labeled antigen bound to the antibody can be calculated.
   c. The concentration of an unknown (unlabeled) antigen can be determined by reference to a standard curve constructed from data obtained by allowing varying amounts of unlabeled antigen to compete.

2. Recent modifications of the previously described liquid-phase RIA involve adsorption or covalent linkage of antibody to a solid matrix (**solid-phase RIA**). Unlabeled antigen is then added, followed by labeled antigen. Determination of bound versus free labeled antigen is then made, and the amount of antigen in the unknown sample is calculated by reference to a standard curve.

3. RIA has wide application in the quantitation of a range of biological substances including:
   a. A number of hormones (e.g., insulin, growth hormone, adrenocorticotropic hormone, triiodothyronine, thyroxine, estrogen)
   b. Serum proteins (e.g., carcinoembryonic antigen, anti-DNA)
   c. Metabolites (e.g., adenosine 3':5'-cyclic phosphate, folic acid)
   d. Drugs (e.g., digoxin, digitoxin, and morphine)
   e. Other microbial agents and antibodies [e.g., hepatitis B surface antigen (HB$_s$Ag)]

H. Enzyme-linked immunosorbent assay (ELISA) has virtually the same sensitivity as RIA.

1. ELISA can be used to assay both antigens and antibodies. The requisites are as follows.
   a. Antigen or antibody can be attached to a **solid-phase support** (e.g., plastic surfaces and paper disks) and still retain its immunologic activity.
   b. Either antigen or antibody can be **linked to an enzyme** (e.g., horseradish peroxidase or alkaline phosphatase) and both immunologic and enzymatic activity are retained by the antigen–enzyme complex.

2. The application of one variant of ELISA, the **double antibody sandwich** for the assay of an antigen (e.g., hepatitis B antigen), is performed as follows.
   a. Antibody specific for the antigen being assayed is coated on a plastic surface (polystyrene

plate). The solution being tested for antigen is applied to the surface, and any unreacted material is removed by washing.

b. Enzyme-labeled specific antibody is then applied, and any excess conjugate is removed by washing. Finally, the enzyme substrate is added.

c. The rate of substrate degradation is determined by the amount of enzyme-labeled antibody bound, which is determined by the amount of antigen in the solution being tested. A substrate that will give a color change on degradation is chosen. The color change can be measured quantitatively in a **spectrophotometer**.

IV. ASSAYS OF IMMUNE COMPETENCE involve evaluating **phagocytic cells, B cells,** and **T cells.**

A. Analysis of phagocytic cells involves three different assays.

1. Assay for metabolism and generation of toxic molecules determines whether phagocytic cells are using the **hexose monophosphate (HMP) shunt** and generating toxic materials to kill microorganisms. It is used in the diagnosis of **chronic granulomatous disease (CGD).** The **nitroblue tetrazolium (NBT) test** is usually used for this assay to determine the phagocytic function of neutrophils.

a. When neutrophils go through the oxidative burst, they reduce the yellow NBT dye to form a dark blue **formazan** precipitate. Cells that do this and contain the formazan precipitate in their cytoplasm are thus formazan-positive (f+) and can be counted. The assay has two parts.

(1) Resting. Dye is placed on the cells, but nothing is administered to trigger oxidation. A normal resting value is 1%–2% f+.

(2) Stimulated. Neutrophils are stimulated to phagocytize. In normal individuals, 100% of the cells can be stimulated to be f+. Patients with CGD lack certain enzymes (e.g., nicotinamide-adenine dinucleotide oxidase) associated with the HMP shunt and therefore do not kill intracellularly; no cells are f+ in either the resting or stimulated states.

b. The NBT test is particularly useful in genetic counseling (CGD is usually an X-linked disease). If the mother is a carrier, she may have 1%–2% f+ in resting neutrophils and an intermediate value when stimulated (e.g., 50%).

2. Assay for ingestion and killing of microorganisms. Some phagocytic disorders are evidenced as a defect in killing, with normal NBT values. In these cases, the **microbicidal assay,** or **intracellular killing assay,** is used in testing the functional integrity of phagocytic cells.

a. In this test, bacteria is added to a tube of neutrophils and incubated for 30 minutes. Enumeration of bacteria inside and outside the cells, with comparison of these numbers to a control with bacteria but no neutrophils, yields a value for percentage of kill. A normal population of cells will kill 85%–90% of the bacteria within 30 minutes.

b. The test can be done by culturing the organisms on suitable bacteriologic media or, alternately, by use of **acridine orange,** a fluorescent dye. Live bacteria will stain green while dead organisms will appear red when observed with a fluorescence microscope.

3. Chemotaxis assay measures the ability of neutrophils to move in a directed, migratory pattern toward stimuli (e.g., complement split products C5a or C5b67). The migration may occur through a nitrocellulose membrane of 3- to 5-μ pore size or in an agar menstruum. The assay must be done in parallel with a normal blood specimen to provide a frame of reference.

B. Analysis of B cells. In all evaluations of immunity, it is important to establish the **number of immune cells** that are present and **whether these cells are functional.** B cells are critical in **humoral immunity,** as are immunoglobulins.

1. Enumeration of cells

a. B cells. Membrane marker assays are used to measure lymphocyte subpopulations. For B cells, the marker is **surface immunoglobulin,** which is an integral membrane component (not just absorbed by a receptor).

(1) The B cells are mixed with an antibody to gamma globulin that has been labeled with **fluorescein dye.**

(2) After incubation, the antibody will have recognized the antigen so that the cell will have fluorescent antibody all around its membrane, which can be detected with a fluorescence microscope.

(3) B cells are identified by their **bright green membrane.**

b. Pre-B cells. The pre-B cell has IgM in its cytoplasm but none on its membrane.

(1) Measurement of pre-B cells is performed by incubating a suspension of viable cells with fluorescein-labeled anti-human μ chain antiserum. The antibody does not enter the cell cytoplasm, but only labels the membrane.

(2) The cells are then washed and fixed on a slide. At this point, the membrane is permeable, and **rhodamine (red)**-labeled anti-human μ serum is added to label any μ chain in the cytoplasm.

(3) Pre-B cells have **cytoplasmic red fluorescence** and no fluorescence on their membranes.

2. **Function**
   a. **Serum immunoglobulin levels.** The quantitation of serum immunoglobulin levels is accomplished by **radial immunodiffusion** (see section II C 3).
   b. **Analysis of serum antibodies.** Some patients have normal immunoglobulin levels but lack specific antibodies. In this case, it must be determined whether the patient can respond to antigens with antibody synthesis. The immunization and past medical history of the patient should be examined prior to deciding which antigen to use.
      (1) Possible antigens include polio virus, tetanus toxoid, diphtheria toxoid, pneumococcal polysaccharide, and **keyhole limpet hemocyanin (KLH)**.
         (a) Since most individuals have had immunizations, they should respond to polio virus, tetanus toxoid, and diphtheria toxoid antigens.
         (b) If the patient has not been immunized, vaccination would be necessary. A killed vaccine should be used; attenuated vaccines can cause infection and death in the immune-deficient patient.
         (c) If an antibody assay of an immunized patient is negative, a **booster injection** could be given, again using killed vaccine.
      (2) In addition, isohemagglutinin levels could be determined to assess B-cell function. Patients in blood group O, A, or B should have anti-A and anti-B, anti-B, or anti-A antibodies, respectively, in their serum by the age of 2 years. If these antibodies are absent, it would indicate a defect in B-cell function.
   c. **Lymphocyte proliferation assays** may also be used to determine the functional status of B cells. The B-cell membrane contains a receptor for lipopolysaccharide (LPS). Interaction of this receptor with LPS will induce mitosis in the lymphocyte. This can be quantitated by determining the amount of radioactive tritium that is incorporated into the DNA of the cell.

C. **Analysis of T cells.** T cells are primarily responsible for **cell-mediated immunity**. The enumeration and function of T cells may be analyzed using the following tests.

1. **Enumeration**
   a. **Erythrocyte rosette (E-rosette) assay** is a marker test for T-cell enumeration.
      (1) If peripheral blood lymphocytes (both T cells and B cells) are mixed with a suspension of SRBCs, the T cells will bind the red blood cells to their membranes and form rosettes (mulberry-shaped cell aggregates); however, B cells do not do this. Since the T cells in their rosette form can now be distinguished from other lymphocytes, they can be enumerated.
      (2) A similar assay, the **erythrocyte–antibody–complement (EAC) rosette test**, can be performed to quantitate B cells if the SRBCs are first coated with antibody and complement.
   b. **T-cell subsets. Fluorescent antibody assays** that utilize monoclonal antibodies to assay specific cell subsets are available. Different monoclonal antibodies interact with different subsets of lymphocytes. Table 8-2 lists the **OKT series** of monoclonal antibodies, the subsets for which they are specific, and the normal values (percent of lymphocytes of that subset in normal blood).

2. **Function**
   a. **Delayed-type hypersensitivity skin testing** is used to test for T-cell function. The procedure in this assay is to conduct a battery of skin tests on the patient in order to evoke a response to one or more antigens. As with serum antibody assays, whether a response occurs depends on what the patient has encountered during his lifetime.

Table 8-2. The Immunologic Specificity of Selected Anti-T–Cell Serums

Antibody*	Subset Detected	Normal Values (%)
OKT 3	Pan-T reagent; reacts with all T cells	75
OKT 4	Helper/inducer T cells	50
OKT 8	Suppressor/cytotoxic T cells	25
OKT 11	All T cells	80

*Recent generic nomenclature updates have changed the OKT series [Ortho Pharmaceuticals] to the CD (cellular differentiation) series [e.g., CD3, CD4, CD8].

     (1) Available antigens include mumps virus, trichophytin (a fungal antigen), candidin (a yeast antigen to which most humans have been exposed), streptokinase–streptodornase (SK-SD, a product of group A β-hemolytic streptococci), purified protein derivative (PPD, a skin test reagent for *Mycobacterium tuberculosis*), and diphtheria toxoid (inactivated toxin from the diphtheria bacillus).

     (2) To perform the test, intradermal injections of the material are given and the patient is observed for the first 3 days after injection.

     (3) A positive test result typically is indicated by an erythematous, indurated lesion that peaks after 48 hours. This reaction is due to the infiltration of cells into the area, which causes it to harden. Usually the erythema is larger than the induration, but **it is the indurated area that is measured**.

   b. Lymphocyte proliferation assays are often used in patient evaluations to determine T-cell function and response to a mitogen [e.g., phytohemagglutinin, concanavalin A, and pokeweed mitogen (mitogenic to both T cells and B cells)].

     (1) The mitogen is mixed with the T cells, which have a specific receptor for the mitogen, causing the T cell to undergo rapid proliferation.

     (2) A radioactive DNA precursor (tritiated thymidine) is used to quantitate the degree of mitosis.

   c. Mixed lymphocyte culture assays depend on the fact that the patient's cells, as the responder, have different histocompatibility antigens on them when compared with target cells drawn from a nonrelated donor.

     (1) The target cells are treated with a drug (e.g., mitomycin C) or irradiation to prevent DNA synthesis and proliferation.

     (2) The patient's responder cells then are mixed with the treated target cells. The patient's cells will recognize the target cells as foreign and should begin proliferation, which can be measured by the addition of tritiated thymidine. If the count is lower than a normal count done on the same day, the patient has **deficient T-cell proliferation**.

V. IDENTIFICATION OF SPECIFIC ALLERGENS IN IMMEDIATE HYPERSENSITIVITY (TYPE I) REACTIONS.

A thorough patient history can be extremely valuable for identification of antigens called **allergens**, particularly if environmental factors are involved. Trial exposure may confirm the etiology; however, precise techniques often must be used.

A. Skin tests involve either cutaneous (scratch test) or intradermal administration of appropriate potential allergens. A positive test is characterized by the appearance of a typical **wheal** (edema) and **flare** (erythema) in the skin within seconds or minutes due to the local release of mediators. Multiple allergens may be tested simultaneously. False-positive and false-negative results are possible. Histamine or a histamine liberator may be administered as a positive control. Antihistaminic drugs must be discontinued 24 hours or more prior to skin testing.

B. Passive transfer tests

   1. Passive cutaneous anaphylaxis (PCA) may be used in experimental animals, such as the guinea pig, to test serum for cytotropic antibody.

     a. Serum is injected intradermally in the shaved skin of a normal animal.

     b. After 3–6 hours, antigen plus Evans blue dye is injected intravenously.

     c. A positive reaction is characterized by bluing of the skin at the injection site due to increased capillary permeability and leakage of dye into the tissues.

   2. The Prausnitz-Küstner (PK) reaction test is comparable to the PCA system described above but is used in humans.

     a. A small amount of serum from an allergic patient, which contains IgE specific for a given allergen, is injected intradermally into a nonallergic person.

     b. The IgE fixes to the skin and mast cells of the recipient during the next 12–24 hours, after which antigenic challenge (i.e., injection of the allergen into the same site) produces a typical wheal and flare reaction.

     c. The PK reaction is not used to any great extent due to the risk of transferring hepatitis and due to the availability of tests that measure total and specific IgE (see below).

C. IgE assays may be used to measure **total IgE levels** as well as **specific IgE levels**.

   1. Radioimmunosorbent test (RIST). This technique is used to measure total IgE concentration.

     a. The serum to be assayed is added to a paper disk—the immunosorbent—to which has been coupled sheep or rabbit antibody to human IgE. The IgE in the serum reacts specifically with the coated disk.

    b. After washing the disk, radiolabeled antibody to human IgE is added to the disk, which couples to the IgE.

    c. After rewashing, the radioactivity of the complex on the disk is measured, the bound radioactivity is directly proportional to the amount of IgE in the serum sample.

  2. Radioallergosorbent test (RAST). This technique is used to measure specific IgE levels.

    a. A specific allergen (e.g., ragweed pollen extract) is coupled to a solid phase, such as a cellulose particle or paper disk. The serum to be examined then is reacted with the solid phase–allergen complex, and if IgE specific for ragweed is present it will fix to the solid phase.

    b. Unbound IgE is removed by washing, after which radiolabeled antibody to human IgE is reacted with the solid phase.

    c. After rewashing, the radioactivity of the particles is measured to give the serum level of IgE specific for ragweed.

VI. DETECTION OF IMMUNE COMPLEXES IN SERUM.
Several assays are available for detecting immune complexes in serum and other biological fluids. These techniques can be divided into three types: solid-phase binding assays, liquid-phase binding assays, and cellular binding assays. An example of each type is given below.

  A. C1q solid-phase binding assay. Complement component C1q has an affinity for immune complexes.

    1. In the solid-phase binding assay, the serum to be tested is incubated in a polystyrene tube that has been coated with C1q. After incubation, the sample is washed out.

    2. The amount of immune complex bound to C1q is quantitated using radiolabeled antibody to immunoglobulin.

  B. C1q liquid-phase binding assay

    1. In the liquid-phase binding assay, radiolabeled C1q is added to the serum being tested.

    2. About 1 hour later, the bound C1q is removed from the free C1q by precipitation with polyethylene glycol.

    3. The amount of radioactivity of the bound C1q corresponds to the C1q binding capacity and indicates the amount of immune complexes.

  C. Raji cell binding assay. This assay is based on the ability of immune complexes to bind Raji cells (a human lymphoblastoid cell line) through C3 receptors. Those cells are well suited for detection of immune complexes because they lack surface immunoglobulin.

    1. Immune complexes bound to the surface of the Raji cells can be assayed by the addition of radiolabeled anti-IgG antibody.

    2. After washing to remove unbound anti-IgG, the cells are quantitated for radioactivity.

STUDY QUESTIONS

Directions: Each question below contains five suggested answers. Choose the **one best** response to each question.

1. In the fluorescent treponemal antibody absorption test used to diagnose syphilis, the patient's serum is added to a slide containing

(A) dead *Treponema pallidum* organisms
(B) fluorescein-tagged antibody to *T. pallidum*
(C) fluorescein-tagged antibody to human gamma globulin
(D) fluorescein isothiocyanate
(E) complement and sheep red blood cells (SRBCs)

2. What is included in the indicator system of a complement fixation test?

(A) Specific antibody and complement
(B) Specific antigen and complement
(C) Red blood cells and hemolysin
(D) Heat-inactivated patient's serum
(E) Guinea pig serum

3. Which of the following tests is the most sensitive measure of antibody?

(A) Precipitation
(B) Agglutination
(C) Radial immunodiffusion
(D) Radioimmunoassay (RIA)
(E) Immunoelectrophoresis

4. In enumerating immune cells, the important marker in the cytoplasm of the pre-B cell is

(A) IgA
(B) IgD
(C) IgE
(D) IgG
(E) IgM

5. In the direct immunofluorescent identification of a specific infectious agent (e.g., *Treponema pallidum* or *Streptococcus pyogenes*), fluorescein may be conjugated to

(A) the microorganism
(B) sheep red blood cells (SRBCs)
(C) antibody specific to human gamma globulin
(D) antibody specific to the microorganism
(E) antibody specific to complement

6. The radioimmunosorbent test (RIST) is a technique used to measure

(A) cellular antigen activity
(B) both antigen and antibody activity
(C) picogram quantities or less of immunogenic or haptenic substances
(D) specific IgE levels
(E) total IgE concentrations

Directions: Each question below contains four suggested answers of which **one or more** is correct. Choose the answer

A   if **1, 2, and 3** are correct
B   if **1 and 3** are correct
C   if **2 and 4** are correct
D   if **4** is correct
E   if **1, 2, 3, and 4** are correct

7. Assays of the functional capability of T cells include

(1) mixed lymphocyte culture
(2) fluorescent antibody assay with T8 antiserum
(3) phytohemagglutinin response
(4) erythrocyte (E) rosette test

8. In order to perform radioimmunoassays (RIAs), it is essential that the substance to be detected

(1) can induce specific antibodies
(2) is protein in nature
(3) can be labeled with a radioactive isotope
(4) does not contain tritiated thymidine

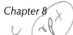

9. The functional integrity of phagocytic cells can be assessed by

(1) microbicidal assay
(2) nitroblue tetrazolium (NBT) test
(3) chemotaxis assay
(4) erythrocyte–antibody–complement (EAC) rosette test

10. Raji cells are well suited for use in an assay used for detection of immune complexes because they lack

(1) bound C1q
(2) free C1q
(3) C3 receptors
(4) surface immunoglobulin

ANSWERS AND EXPLANATIONS

1. The answer is A. (*III B 2 a*) Direct and indirect immunofluorescence techniques use fluorescent dyes, such as fluorescein isothiocyanate, to conjugate to antibody molecules in order to identify antigens. One type of indirect immunofluorescence is the fluorescent treponemal antibody absorption test, which detects antibodies to *Treponema pallidum*, the etiologic agent of syphilis. *T. pallidum* fixed to a slide is flooded with the patient's serum. These antibodies react with the spirochetes on the slide, which are subsequently visualized by the use of a fluorescent microscope and fluorescein-labeled anti-human gamma globulin.

2. The answer is C. (*III A 2 a, c*) The test system contains antibody and/or antigen and complement (e.g., guinea pig serum). To ascertain whether complement has been fixed (consumed), it is necessary to add a second set of reagents, the indicator system, which must react to the presence of active complement in a visible way. The indicator system consists of sheep red blood cells (SRBCs) plus antibody (hemolysin) specific for SRBCs. The SRBCs will be lysed if they are first sensitized to complement lysis by anti-SRBC antibody, such as hemolysin.

3. The answer is D. (*III G; Table 8-1*) Radioimmunoassay (RIA) and enzyme-linked immunosorbent assay (ELISA) are the most sensitive of methods available for the detection of antigens and antibodies. Precipitation is among the least sensitive tests, followed by (in order of increasing sensitivity) immuno-electrophoresis, radial immunodiffusion, and bacterial agglutination. Table 8-1 provides further listing of the sensitivity of various serologic procedures.

4. The answer is E. [*IV B 1 b (1) (2)*] The pre-B cell has IgM in its cytoplasm but none on its membrane. Pre-B cells are enumerated by incubating a suspension of viable cells with fluorescein-labeled anti-human μ chain antiserum. At this point, the antibody is unable to enter the cell cytoplasm but it can label the membrane. After the cells are washed and fixed on a slide, the membrane is permeable, and rhodamine (red)-labeled anti-human μ serum is added to label any μ chain in the cytoplasm.

5. The answer is D. (*III B 1*) In direct immunofluorescence, the fluorescein is conjugated directly onto the antibody that will react with the specific pathogen. Fluorescein-tagged anti-human gamma globulin is used in indirect tests. Some procedures employ two labeled antibodies—one fluorescein-conjugated and a second labeled with rhodamine, which fluoresces red. Thus, different cellular structures, or organisms, can be visualized at the same time.

6. The answer is E. (*V C 1*) The radioimmunosorbent test (RIST) is an assay used to measure total IgE concentration, and is useful in identifying specific allergens in immediate hypersensitivity (type I) reactions. Specific IgE levels are measured by the radioallergosorbent test (RAST). Cellular antigen activity is identified using agglutination reactions. Radioimmunoassay (RIA) is used to quantitate picogram quantities or less of substances that are immunogenic or haptenic and can be labeled with a radioactive isotope. The enzyme-linked immunosorbent assay (ELISA) is used to assay both antigens and antibodies using solid-phase support and enzyme linking as requisites.

7. The answer is B (1, 3). (*IV C 1 a, b, 2 b, c*) The mixed lymphocyte culture, fluorescent antibody assay with T8 antiserum, phytohemagglutinin response, and erythrocyte (E) rosette test, all will measure some T-cell characteristic. Only the mixed lymphocyte culture and phytohemagglutinin response, however, will reflect the functional status of the cells. T8 is the membrane marker seen on suppressor and cytotoxic T cells. E-rosettes are formed by T cells when they are mixed with sheep red blood cells.

8. The answer is B (1, 3). (*III G*) In order to successfully perform radioimmunoassays, it is a prerequisite that the material being assayed be immunogenic, since an essential ingredient in the procedure is specific antibody. Further, the substance must be able to be labeled with radioactive materials without undergoing any immunologic alterations that would interfere in its reactivity with its homologous antibody. The radioactivity of the antigen is immaterial as it would be subtracted as background and/or would not be detected in the assay. For example, an antigen containing tritiated thymidine would not emit gamma rays and hence would not be confused with the ^{125}I content of the sample being evaluated.

9. The answer is A (1, 2, 3). [*IV A 1, 2, 3, C 1 a (2)*] Intracellular destruction of bacteria can be measured by the microbicidal assay. The nitroblue tetrazolium (NBT) test measures hexose monophosphate shunt activity that occurs during phagocytosis. Chemotactic responsiveness is an important attribute of phagocytic cells, which is usually measured by enumerating cells that have migrated through a membrane. The erythrocyte–antibody–complement (EAC) rosette assay is a measure of the number of B cells in a specimen. B cells have membrane receptors for the Fc portion of antibody as well as a receptor for C3b, and hence will react with erythrocytes coated with these molecules.

10. The answer is D (4). (*VI C*) Raji cell binding assay is based on the ability of immune complexes to bind to Raji cells, a human lymphoblastoid cell line, through C3 receptors. Raji cells are well suited for detection of immune complexes because they lack surface immunoglobulin. When bound to the surface of the Raji cells, immune complexes can be assayed by the addition of radiolabeled anti-IgG antibody.

9

Immunologic Mechanisms of Tissue Damage

I. INTRODUCTION

A. Hypersensitivity reactions. Although the immune system generally is protective, the same immunologic mechanisms that defend the host at times may result in severe damage to tissues and, occasionally, may cause death. Gell and Coombs have classified these damaging immunologic reactions (also called hypersensitivity reactions) into four major types: immediate hypersensitivity (type I) reactions, cytotoxic (type II) reactions, immune complex-mediated (type III) reactions, and delayed hypersensitivity (cell-mediated, type IV) reactions.

B. Plasma cell dyscrasias (also called paraproteinemias or monoclonal gammopathies) are diseases that are characterized by the overproduction of immunoglobulins or their fragments by a single clone of plasma cells; the protein is called a paraprotein. Plasma cell dyscrasias also may cause tissue damage and are discussed in section VI.

II. IMMEDIATE HYPERSENSITIVITY REACTIONS

A. Definition. Immediate hypersensitivity reactions are initiated by antigens reacting with cell-bound antibody, usually IgE. The immediate hypersensitivity may manifest in many ways, depending on the target organ or tissue, and may range from life-threatening anaphylactic reactions to the lesser annoyances of atopic allergies (e.g., hay fever and food allergies).

B. Pathogenic mechanism. Immediate hypersensitivity reactions involve the release of pharmacologically active substances, or mediators, from mast cells or basophils, a mechanism which is triggered by antigens reacting with preformed, cell-bound IgE molecules.

1. Allergens are antigens that induce production of specific IgE antibodies in humans. Allergens include such diverse substances as:
  a. Plant pollens (e.g., ragweed) and mold spores (e.g., *Alternaria* and *Aspergillus*)
  b. House dust, the most likely antigenic component of which is the **house dust mite**
  c. Animal hair, dander, and feathers
  d. Foods (e.g., milk, wheat, eggs, fish, and chocolate)
  e. Foreign serums and hormones
  f. Insect venoms (e.g., bee and wasp)
  g. Drugs and chemicals (e.g., antibiotics, antiseptics, anesthetics, and vitamins)

2. IgE antibody (reagin). Although other immunoglobulin classes have been implicated in immediate hypersensitivity reactions in animals (including humans), the primary antibody responsible for such reactivity in humans in IgE.
  a. Structural and chemical properties of IgE are discussed in Chapter 3, section III E.
  b. IgE production
    (1) IgE is produced by plasma cells in the spleen, lymphoid tissues, and mucosa of the respiratory and gastrointestinal tracts. IgE production may occur following initial contact with a specific allergen.
    (2) Regulation of IgE production appears to be independent of IgG, IgM, and IgA responses. Experimental studies in animals suggest that IgE production is firmly under the control of IgE-specific T cells, which can produce both IgE-potentiating and IgE-suppressing factors.

3. Mediators. If the initial exposure to an allergen results in the production of specific IgE, with its ultimate fixation to cells, subsequent exposure to the allergen triggers an antigen–antibody reaction on the cell membrane. Bridging of adjacent membrane-bound IgE molecules by specific antigen (allergen) initiates degranulation and release of mediators stored in mast cells and basophils. Mediator release requires energy and appears to be modulated by such cellular energy sources as calcium (Ca^{2+}), proesterase, esterase, cyclic adenosine $3',5'$-monophosphate (cAMP), and cyclic guanosine $3',5'$-monophosphate (cGMP).

    a. Histamine probably is the most important mediator. It causes smooth muscle contraction and increased capillary permeability as well as increased nasal secretions and airway resistance. Histamine exists preformed in mast cells and basophils and is released upon degranulation.

    b. Slow-reacting substance of anaphylaxis (SRS-A) does not exist preformed in mediator cells; its production is induced by the antigen-antibody reaction. SRS-A, a leukotriene, is a lipoxygenase metabolite of arachidonic acid. Like histamine, SRS-A contracts smooth muscle and increases capillary permeability, but it does so in a more prolonged manner. Probably it is a major factor in the bronchospasm that occurs in asthma.

    c. Bradykinin is a nonapeptide (a chain of 9 amino acids), which is derived from serum α_2-macroglobulin through the action of the enzyme kallikrein. It causes smooth muscle contraction in a slow, prolonged manner, increases vascular permeability, and increases mucus secretion by mucous glands.

    d. Serotonin (5-hydroxytryptamine) appears to be an important mediator of anaphylaxis in animals other than humans. It exists in a preformed state and, when released, causes smooth muscle contraction and increased capillary permeability.

    e. Eosinophil chemotactic factor of anaphylaxis (ECF-A) exists in a preformed state as an acidic peptide and has a molecular weight of about 500. It attracts eosinophils to areas of allergic inflammation. Eosinophils exert feedback control on allergic reactions through their release of arylsulfatase B, which inactivates SRS-A, and histaminase, which inactivates histamine.

    f. Platelet activating factor (PAF) is an acetyl glyceryl ether phosphorylcholine that does not exist preformed but is generated by the antigen-antibody reaction. It causes platelet aggregation and release of vasoactive amines, leading to increased vascular permeability, smooth muscle contraction, and bronchoconstriction. In skin, PAF produces a wheal and flare reaction that is not blocked by antihistamines. PAF is inactivated by phospholipases.

    g. Prostaglandins are products of cyclooxygenase metabolism of arachidonic acid. Prostaglandin E_1 (PGE_1) and PGE_2 are potent bronchodilators and vasodilators. PGI_2 (also called prostacyclin) disaggregates platelets.

  4. Genetic factors appear to play a role in atopic allergies (see section II C 2). Hay fever, asthma, and food allergies, for example, show familial tendency; there is a strong probability that children of two atopic parents will also be atopic. The IgE response to allergens seems to be associated with specific human leukocyte antigens (HLAs). A subtle defect in suppressor T (Ts) cells is thought to lead to the increased IgE response in the atopic individual.

C. Clinical features leading to a diagnosis (see Chapter 8, section V) of immediate hypersensitivity reactions vary greatly in severity and character, depending on the target organ or tissue and whether the condition is anaphylactic or atopic.

  1. Anaphylaxis refers to an immediate hypersensitivity response that is inducible in a normal host of any given species upon appropriate antigenic exposure (called sensitization).

    a. The response may be either systemic (anaphylactic shock) or local but in all species is primarily characterized by smooth muscle contraction and increased capillary permeability.

    b. The primary target organ, or **shock organ**, varies from species to species; examples include the lung (in guinea pigs and humans), the heart (in rabbits), and the liver (in dogs). The immediate hypersensitivity response in the guinea pig is a classic presentation of convulsions, itching, sneezing, urination, defecation, and death (within minutes) due to severe bronchoconstriction and trapping of air in the lungs.

  2. Atopy refers to an immediate hypersensitivity response that occurs only in genetically predisposed hosts upon sensitization to specific allergens. This condition differs from anaphylaxis in that it cannot be induced in normal hosts. The strong hereditary association noted in atopic allergies was once thought to be restricted to humans but has been described in other animal species.

    a. As in anaphylactic reactions, the response in atopic reactions is characterized by smooth muscle contraction and increased capillary permeability.

    b. Specific types of atopic reactions include bronchial asthma, allergic rhinitis (hay fever), urticaria (hives) and angioedema, and atopic dermatitis (eczema).

D. Therapy

  1. Avoidance. The most direct way to manage allergic disease is through environmental control;

that is, avoidance of the specific allergen(s) responsible for the allergic reaction. This can be accomplished quite easily with food allergies but may be difficult with inhalant allergies.

2. Hyposensitization is a form of immunotherapy aimed at stimulating the production of IgG blocking antibody, which binds the offending allergen and prevents its combining with IgE.

3. Administration of modified allergens, or "allergoids," is a form of immunotherapy aimed at stimulating production of IgG blocking antibody as well as IgE-specific Ts cells.

4. Drug treatment involves administration of agents designed to:
  a. Block mediators from binding to target tissue (e.g., diphenhydramine)
  b. Stabilize lysosomal membranes (e.g., corticosteroids)
  c. Stimulate adenyl cyclase, the enzyme responsible for conversion of adenosine triphosphate (ATP) to cAMP and, thereby, block the release of mediators (e.g., epinephrine)
  d. Block the release of mediators by stabilizing mast cell membranes (e.g., sodium cromolyn)
  e. Inhibit phosphodiesterase, an enzyme that converts cAMP to AMP, thus preserving levels of cAMP essential for blockage of mediator release (e.g., theophylline)

III. CYTOTOXIC REACTIONS

A. Definition. Cytotoxic reactions are initiated by antibody—usually IgG or IgM—reacting with cell-bound antigen.

B. Pathogenic mechanism. Cytotoxic reactions involve primarily either the combination of IgG or IgM antibodies with epitopes on cell surface or tissue or the adsorption of antigens or haptens to tissue or cell membrane, with subsequent attachment of antibodies to the adsorbed antigens. Either mechanism may lead to one of the following destructive processes.

1. Activation of complement, with subsequent lysis or inactivation of target cells

2. Phagocytosis of target cells, with or without complement activation

3. Lysis or inactivation of target cells via effector lymphoid cells (e.g., ADCC)

C. Clinical features. The many types of cytotoxic reactions can be grouped according to the nature of the target cell or tissue damage that occurs in the reaction.

1. Red blood cell lysis probably is the most important clinical phenomenon associated with cytotoxic reactions. The following are classic examples.
  a. Transfusion reactions may be classified as immunologic or nonimmunologic. Immunologically mediated transfusion reactions may occur by two different mechanisms: rapid intravascular destruction of transfused red blood cells or extravascular destruction of antibody-sensitized red blood cells, primarily by the reticuloendothelial system (RES).
    (1) Intravascular hemolysis of red blood cells usually is associated with **ABO system incompatibility.** The ABO blood group system consists of gene loci that are specific for antigens appearing on the red blood cell surface. Because antibodies to the ABO system occur naturally, it is important to match donor blood to recipient blood, as blood transfusion into a person who has antibodies to those red blood cells can produce a transfusion reaction. This reaction is characterized by erythrocyte-bound anti-A or anti-B antibodies activating complement, with almost immediate lysis of transfused red blood cells.
    (2) Extravascular hemolysis of red blood cells almost invariably is associated with Rh incompatibility. The Rh blood group system consists of several distinct Rh antigens, which exist on the red blood cell membrane and strongly stimulate antibody formation when introduced into the blood of persons who lack these antigens. The Rh antigen most commonly involved is $Rh_0(D)$. Unlike anti-A and anti-B antibodies, anti-Rh antibodies do not cause complement-mediated intravascular hemolysis. Instead, there is antibody-mediated adhesion and phagocytosis of sensitized red blood cells by peripheral blood granulocytes, monocytes, and macrophages.
    (3) Symptoms of transfusion reactions include fever, back pain, chills, malaise, hypotension, nausea, and vomiting. These manifestations are more pronounced in reactions that are due to intravascular hemolysis than in those due to extravascular hemolysis. Acute renal failure is a serious complication of intravascular hemolytic transfusion reactions.
    (4) Prevention of transfusion reactions includes careful blood-typing and cross-matching.
  b. Hemolytic disease of the newborn
    (1) Etiology and pathogenesis
      (a) Hemolytic disease of the newborn (erythroblastosis fetalis) occurs when an Rh-neg-

ative mother gives birth to an Rh-positive infant, the Rh antigen having been acquired from an Rh-positive father. The most commonly involved antigen is $Rh_0(D)$.

   (b) In order for this condition to occur, the mother must be sensitized to blood group antigens of the infant's red blood cells. Sensitization may occur during pregnancy, if fetal blood leaks into the maternal circulation (a small amount of transplacental blood leakage is normal). However, the major risk occurs during delivery, when large amounts of cord blood enter the mother's circulation.

   (c) After sensitization, IgG antibodies to the $Rh_0(D)$ antigen are produced, which may cross the placenta and destroy fetal cells. The first child usually is not affected, but the chance sensitization increases with subsequent pregnancies.

   (2) Symptoms noted in affected infants include anemia and jaundice, which usually develop during the first 24 hours of life; hepatosplenomegaly; and bilirubin encephalopathy (in untreated infants).

   (3) Management. In severe cases, infants require exchange transfusion.

   (4) Prevention of Rh hemolytic disease of the newborn is accomplished best by preventing maternal sensitization to fetal Rh antigens or inhibiting production of antibodies to those antigens. The administration of anti-Rh antibodies Rh_0 IgG (RhoGAM) to an Rh-negative mother within 72 hours of delivering an Rh-positive infant will prevent sensitization and problems with subsequent pregnancies, probably via rapid destruction and clearance of Rh-positive cells from the circulation [see Chapter 6, section II B 2 c (2)].

   c. **Autoimmune hemolytic disease.** Warm antibody hemolytic anemia, cold antibody hemolytic anemia, and paroxysmal cold hemoglobinuria are discussed in Chapter 10, section V K.

   2. **White blood cell lysis**

   a. **Systemic lupus erythematosus (SLE)** [see Chapter 10, section V H] is characterized by the presence of several antibodies in the serum, including antinuclear antibodies, antibodies to membrane and cytoplasmic components, and antibodies cytotoxic to blood cellular elements (i.e., lymphocytes, platelets, and red blood cells). [SLE can be considered a mixed disease (both types II and III).]

   b. **Granulocytopenia.** Cytotoxic reactions involving antibodies to neutrophils or to drugs adsorbed to neutrophil surfaces can result in granulocytopenia and a consequent phagocytic defect, leading to increased susceptibility to infection.

   c. **Idiopathic thrombocytopenic purpura (ITP)** [see Chapter 10, section V L] is characterized by the presence of IgG antibodies specific for platelets, which can lead to various bleeding disorders.

   3. **Nephrotoxic nephritis** is an experimental glomerulonephritis that can be induced in rats by injection of heterologous antibodies against glomerular basement membrane or by active immunization with antigens isolated from glomerular basement membrane. The disease is characterized by proteinuria, impaired glomerular filtration, neutrophil infiltration of glomeruli, and antibody deposition in a linear pattern along the glomerular basement membrane, which is visible on immunofluorescent imaging. A similar clinical picture is seen in humans and is referred to as Goodpasture's syndrome (see Chapter 10, section V M).

   4. **Bullous diseases** (e.g., pemphigus vulgaris and bullous pemphigoid; see Chapter 10, section V O) are characterized by antibody and complement deposition in squamous intercellular spaces and along the basement membrane of the skin.

D. **Therapy** for cytotoxic reactions includes treatment of the underlying cause of the reaction as well as the subsequent manifestations of such a reaction. Examples of therapeutic measures include:

   1. **Suppression of the immune response** by means of corticosteroids, with or without cytotoxic immunosuppressive drugs (e.g., cyclophosphamide and azathioprine) or by splenectomy

   2. **Removal of offending antibodies** via exchange transfusion (in the case of Rh hemolytic disease of the newborn) or plasmapheresis (in the case of Goodpasture's syndrome)

   3. **Withholding the offending drug** (in the case of a drug-induced syndrome such as ITP)

   4. **Nephrectomy** (in the case of Goodpasture's syndrome)

IV. IMMUNE COMPLEX-MEDIATED REACTIONS

A. **Definition.** Immune complex-mediated reactions are initiated by antigen–antibody (immune) complexes that either are formed locally (at the site of tissue damage) or are deposited from the circulation. Immune complex disorders are characterized by the presence of antigen–antibody complexes in vascular and glomerular basement membranes.

B. Pathogenic mechanism. The pathogenesis of immune complex disorders involves an interplay of antigen, antibody, complement, and neutrophils.

   1. The first step is the formation of soluble immune complexes, which generally occurs in the region of antigen excess. Virtually any antigen that induces a detectable antibody response will serve. In addition to the antigens described in section IV C, the following microbial antigens also should be cited: *Treponema pallidum*, *Plasmodium* species, Epstein-Barr virus (EBV), hepatitis B virus, and *Mycobacterium leprae*. The antibodies involved are primarily precipitating IgG and IgM capable of fixing complement.

   2. Being soluble, the immune complexes escape phagocytosis, penetrate the endothelium of blood vessel walls (probably with the aid of vasoactive amines released from platelets and basophils), and are deposited on the vascular basement membrane.

   3. Complement is activated with the release of factors that are chemotactic for neutrophils (i.e., C5a and C5b67); the neutrophils then infiltrate the area and release lysosomal enzymes that destroy the basement membrane.

C. Clinical features. The following are classic examples of immune complex-mediated reactions.

   1. Arthus reaction. This necrotic dermal reaction is considered to be a local immune complex-deposition phenomenon, which is observed in rabbits that have been repeatedly injected subcutaneously with antigen (i.e., normal horse serum). The rabbits tolerate the first few doses without any local reactions; however, the injections induce the formation of antibodies specific for horse serum proteins. With subsequent exposures, foci of erythema, edema, and necrosis are noted at the injection sites. Microscopic examination of tissue reveals accumulation of neutrophils plus a vasculitis related to destruction of the basement membrane of blood vessel walls. The Arthus reaction was observed first in rabbits; similar reactions are observed in other animals, including humans.

   2. Serum sickness refers to the syndrome that follows the injection of foreign serum into humans. Considered to be a **systemic immune complex-deposition phenomenon**, serum sickness first was seen following the administration of diphtheria antitoxin (prepared in horses) to humans. The syndrome is characterized by fever, rash, splenomegaly, lymphadenopathy, arthritis, and glomerulonephritis.* As is noted in the Arthus reaction, the primary damage observed in serum sickness appears to be a vasculitis associated with destruction of vascular basement membrane.

   3. Hypersensitivity pneumonitis (also called **extrinsic allergic alveolitis**) refers to the lung parenchymal reaction to repeated inhalation of organic dusts, such as thermophilic actinomycetes (**farmer's lung, bagassosis**), mold spores (**malt worker's lung**), and fragments of avian matter (**bird breeder's lung**).
   a. Pathogenesis. Patients often have antibodies to the offending substances, with deposition of antigen–antibody complexes in target (lung) tissue; this suggests a type III reaction. Recent evidence suggests that, in addition to immune complexes, type IV (delayed hypersensitivity) reactions also play a role in the pathogenesis of hypersensitivity pneumonitis.
   b. Symptoms include fever, chills, chest pain, cough, and dyspnea, which occur 4–8 hours after exposure. In severe, chronic cases, irreversible lung damage (fibrosis) may occur.

   4. Poststreptococcal glomerulonephritis is an immune complex glomerulonephritis characterized by proteinuria and hematuria and red blood cell casts in urine. Antibody, complement, and bacterial antigen are present in the renal vasculature.

   5. Autoimmune disease. Endogenous antigen–antibody–complement complexes are involved in the pathogenesis of certain autoimmune diseases, such as rheumatoid arthritis and SLE.

D. Therapy for immune complex-mediated reactions includes:

   1. Suppression of immune response by means of corticosteroids and cytotoxic immunosuppressive drugs (e.g., cyclophosphamide, azathioprine)

   2. Removal of offending complexes via plasmapheresis

V. DELAYED HYPERSENSITIVITY REACTIONS

A. Definition. Delayed hypersensitivity reactions are initiated by sensitized (antigen-reactive) T cells

*The hallmark of immune complex glomerulonephritis is its granular ("lumpy, bumpy") appearance as detected by direct immunofluorescence using tagged antibody specific for immunoglobulin or complement. In this way, immune complex glomerulonephritis can be differentiated from autoimmune or idiopathic injury to the glomerular basement membrane, in which a smooth, linear pattern of immunoglobulin deposition is observed.

reacting with specific antigens. The reactions manifest as inflammation at the site of antigen exposure, which usually peaks 24–48 hours after exposure.

B. Pathogenic mechanism. Delayed hypersensitivity (cell-mediated) tissue damage results from the interaction between sensitized T cells and specific antigen, which leads to the release of soluble effector substances called lymphokines, direct cytotoxicity, or both. This reaction is independent of antibody and complement but is dependent upon two types of functioning T cells: **T4 + cells** [a population of effector T (Te or T$_{DTH}$) cells for delayed hypersensitivity and cells that help to produce cytotoxic/suppressor cells] and **T8 + cells** (a population of cytotoxic cells and suppressor cells).

1. **Transfer of delayed hypersensitivity.** Cell-mediated immunity can be transferred from a sensitized animal to a nonsensitized animal (including humans) with antigen-reactive T cells; it cannot be transferred passively with serum containing antibodies. Another mechanism for the transfer of delayed hypersensitivity is by a small molecule called **transfer factor**, a dialyzable extract of leukocytes (see Chapter 7, section V B 13).

2. **Mediators of delayed hypersensitivity.** The first step in the delayed hypersensitivity reaction is binding of antigen to specific antigen-reactive T cells (see section V B 3). The antigen triggers the T cells to produce and release various lymphokines, which have many different biological activities. It is not known how many biochemically distinct lymphokines exist; however, the following are among those generally recognized.
   a. **Migration inhibition factor (MIF)** inhibits migration of macrophages.
   b. **Macrophage activation factor (MAF)** enhances microbicidal and cytolytic activity of macrophages.
   c. **Macrophage chemotactic factor** stimulates infiltration of macrophages.
   d. **Transfer factor**
   e. **Leukocyte inhibition factor (LIF)** inhibits random migration of neutrophils.
   f. **Interleukin-2** stimulates growth of activated T cells; it is a mitogenic factor.
   g. **Lymphotoxin** has the ability to lyse certain tumor cells.
   h. **Gamma interferon** functions similarly to MAF.

3. **Induction of delayed hypersensitivity.** These reactions are induced by the uptake of antigen by macrophages and the activation of T cells. Induction requires that the T cells recognize immunogenic epitopes as well as determinants in the major histocompatibility complex (MHC) gene products.
   a. Interaction between antigen-processing cells and T cells can occur only if the two participants are MHC identical (see Chapter 5, section V A 2 a–c and Chapter 12, section II).
      (1) The T4+ cell population contains effector cells for delayed hypersensitivity, which recognize antigen in conjunction with class II molecules (e.g., HLA-DR).
      (2) The T8+ cell population contains cytotoxic/suppressor cells, which recognize antigen in conjunction with class I molecules (e.g., HLA-A, HLA-B, HLA-C). T4+ cells aid in the development of T8+ cells by generating interleukin-2 and possibly other factors.
   b. Under the influence of antigen and MHC gene products, one of two types of antigen-reactive (sensitized) cells is produced.
      (a) Effector cells are capable of passive transfer of sensitivity and release of effector lymphokines.
      (b) Cytotoxic T (Tc) cells are capable—directly or indirectly (via lymphokines)—of killing target cells (e.g., grafted tissue, tumors, and virus-infected cells).

C. Clinical features

1. Delayed hypersensitivity plays a critical role in **cell-mediated immunity**.
   a. As a result, delayed hypersensitivity reactions provide resistance to:
      (1) Chronic intracellular **bacterial infections** (e.g., tuberculosis and brucellosis)
      (2) **Fungal infections** (e.g., blastomycosis and histoplasmosis)
      (3) **Viral infections** (e.g., herpes and mumps)
      (4) **Protozoan infections** (e.g., leishmaniasis)
      (5) **Tumors** (although cytotoxic antibody also may be involved)
   b. As another expression of cell-mediated immunity, delayed hypersensitivity also plays a role in the **rejection of grafted tissues and organs**. (Humoral immunity also may be involved in allograft rejection.)
   c. Finally, delayed hypersensitivity reactions provide the basic mechanism of tissue injury in a variety of diseases, such as:
      (1) **Contact dermatitis**, a delayed hypersensitivity reaction that occurs in response to antigen exposure on skin

(2) **Autoimmune diseases** (e.g., Hashimoto's thyroiditis)

2. The classic example of delayed hypersensitivity is demonstrated by the **tuberculin skin test reaction**.
   a. A small amount of antigen—usually purified protein derivative of tuberculin (PPD)—is injected intradermally into an appropriately sensitized person.
   b. The reaction appears slowly, about 12–24 hours after the injection, and reaches maximal reactivity 24–48 hours later. Initially, there is erythema and a neutrophil infiltrate; later, a mononuclear cell (lymphocyte and macrophage) infiltrate causes induration in the region of the injection.

D. **Modulation of delayed hypersensitivity.** Numerous agents have been shown to affect delayed hypersensitivity, either by suppressing or enhancing reactivity.

1. **Suppressant agents**
   a. **Corticosteroids** (e.g., cortisone) suppress the inflammatory response through their effect on lymphocytes; that is, lymphocytes are redistributed to the bone marrow and intravascular space.
   b. **Antilymphocyte**, or **antithymocyte**, **serum** depletes lymphocyte numbers via direct cytotoxicity.
   c. **Cytotoxic immunosuppressive drugs** (e.g., azathioprine, cyclosporine, and cyclophosphamide) often are employed to control organ rejection after transplantation.

2. **Enhancing agents**
   a. **Thymic hormones**, such as thymosin and thymopoietin, promote the development of immunocompetent T cells and T-cell differentiation, respectively.
   b. **Levamisole** has been shown to be an immunostimulating agent in experimental animals and humans, although it is not approved for use in humans in the United States. The drug appears to restore cell-mediated immune mechanisms of peripheral leukocytes and also may enhance macrophage–T-cell interaction and macrophage activity.
   c. **Isoprinosine** is an experimental antiviral agent that has been shown to enhance T-cell function and macrophage activity. This drug has not been approved for use in humans in the United States.

E. **Cutaneous basophil hypersensitivity** refers to a group of delayed-onset, T-cell–mediated reactions that have been experimentally induced in animals as well as in humans. These reactions mimic delayed hypersensitivity reactions in that they are T-cell–mediated and transferred passively with lymphocytes; however, they differ in a few significant ways. For example, basophils comprise 50% of the cell exudate, the lesions lack the induration seen in classic delayed hypersensitivity reactions, and cutaneous basophil hypersensitivity usually is seen soon after immunization and is short-lived.

VI. **PLASMA CELL DYSCRASIAS** represent a group of diseases characterized by the overproduction of immunoglobulins, or their fragments, by a single clone of plasma cells. The protein is called **paraprotein**. The most important of the plasma cell dyscrasias is multiple myeloma; other notable disorders include Waldenström's macroglobulinemia, benign monoclonal gammopathy, primary amyloidosis, and heavy chain diseases.

A. **Multiple myeloma** is a plasma cell tumor in bone marrow that overproduces a single class of immunoglobulin; most cases involve IgG.

1. The most characteristic feature of multiple myeloma is the demonstration of an abnormal protein (**M protein**) in the blood, urine, or both. The M protein usually consists of any one or a combination of heavy chains, IgG, IgA, and light chains. In some cases (about 10%), a substance called **Bence-Jones protein** (a dimer of light chains) is found in the urine (pyroglobulinuria). When the urine is heated to 50°–60°C, the protein precipitates; upon boiling, it dissolves.

2. The clinical features and complications of multiple myeloma vary widely. Some of the more common manifestations include:
   a. Bone pain and pathologic fractures
   b. Bone marrow infiltration by an abundance of abnormal plasma cells, with resultant normochromic normocytic anemia
   c. Renal abnormalities, possibly resulting in chronic renal failure
   d. Fatigue and weakness

B. **Waldenström's macroglobulinemia** is a lymphocytic lymphoma characterized by overproduction of lymphocytes, plasma cells, and lymphocytes that resemble plasma cells.

1. The most distinguishing feature of this disorder is a high level of monoclonal IgM in the serum. Bence-Jones proteins also may be seen in the urine.

2. Because of the high serum IgM, patients have a hyperviscosity of the blood, which may be severe. Anemia, lymphadenopathy, and chronic lymphocytic leukemia also are common clinical features.

C. **Benign monoclonal gammopathy** refers to a condition seen in older persons (usually older than age 70 years) who are otherwise normal but reveal an increased serum concentration of monoclonal protein—usually IgG, but occasionally IgM. There usually are no other manifestations of disease. However, some patients are at risk for developing multiple myeloma.

D. **Amyloidosis** is a disease characterized by deposition of an abnormal protein (amyloid) in the vascular endothelium of various organs of the body. The clinical features seen in amyloidosis patients depend on the site and extent of amyloid deposition. Two types of amyloidosis have been defined.

1. **Primary amyloidosis** is a plasma cell dyscrasia characterized by the accumulation of amyloid fibrils that are composed primarily of immunoglobulin light chain fragments. This type of amyloidosis often is associated with multiple myeloma.

2. **Secondary amyloidosis** refers to amyloidosis that occurs in the context of chronic infection or inflammation. The amyloid fibrils in secondary amyloidosis bear no structural resemblance to those seen in primary amyloidosis and are called "**AA proteins.**"

E. **Heavy chain diseases** are rare malignancies characterized by a serum paraprotein consisting of incomplete heavy chains without light chains. The abnormal heavy chain structurally is characterized by partial deletion of the Fd portion, deletion of the hinge region, or a combination of both abnormalities. Gamma, alpha, and mu heavy chain diseases have been described.

F. **Therapy** for plasma cell dyscrasias includes such techniques as:

1. Administration of prednisone, with or without cytotoxic drugs (e.g., melphalan and cyclophosphamide)

2. Removal of excess protein (e.g., IgM in Waldenström's macroglobulinemia) via plasmapheresis

STUDY QUESTIONS

Directions: Each question below contains five suggested answers. Choose the **one best** response to each question.

1. Immunotherapy for atopy induces formation of which of the following blocking antibodies?

(A) IgA
(B) IgD
(C) IgE
(D) IgG
(E) IgM

2. The pathogenesis of immune complex disorders involves an interplay of antigen, antibody, neutrophils, and which of the following complement-derived factors?

(A) C$\overline{1}$s
(B) Cla4b
(C) C3b inactivator
(D) C3 activator
(E) C5a

3. Lymphokines play a mediator role in the manifestation of which of the following hypersensitivities?

(A) Delayed hypersensitivity
(B) Serum sickness
(C) Atopy
(D) Hemolytic disease of the newborn
(E) Anaphylaxis

4. Epinephrine is valuable in the management of atopy through its ability to block mediator release by

(A) inhibiting phosphodiesterase
(B) inhibiting production of histamine
(C) inhibiting slow-reacting substance of anaphylaxis (SRS-A)
(D) stimulating production of adenyl cyclase
(E) stimulating release of lymphokines

5. What is the major protein component of the amyloid deposits seen in patients with primary amyloidosis?

(A) Complement protein fragments
(B) Intact IgM
(C) Immunoglobulin light chain fragments
(D) Aggregated IgG
(E) IgE heavy chain

6. Which of the following disorders is characterized by overproduction of monoclonal IgG?

(A) Serum sickness
(B) Acquired immune deficiency syndrome (AIDS)
(C) Waldenström's macroglobulinemia
(D) Hypersensitivity pneumonitis
(E) Multiple myeloma

Directions: Each question below contains four suggested answers of which **one or more** is correct. Choose the answer

A if **1, 2, and 3** are correct
B if **1 and 3** are correct
C if **2 and 4** are correct
D if **4** is correct
E if **1, 2, 3, and 4** are correct

7. The pharmacologically active mediators of anaphylaxis include

(1) serotonin
(2) histamine
(3) bradykinin
(4) platelet-activating factor (PAF)

8. Delayed hypersensitivity (cell-mediated; type IV) reactions are suppressed by

(1) macrophage depletion
(2) complement depletion
(3) cortisone
(4) antihistamines

SUMMARY OF DIRECTIONS

A	B	C	D	E
1, 2, 3 only	1, 3 only	2, 4 only	4 only	All are correct

9. The pathogenetic requirements for immune complex-induced glomerulonephritis include

(1) red blood cell and complement interaction
(2) neutrophil activity
(3) kidney-derived antigen
(4) small, soluble immune complexes

10. Allergic urticaria is best described as being a manifestation of

(1) delayed hypersensitivity
(2) an immunodeficiency disorder
(3) an autoimmune disorder
(4) an IgE-mediated disorder

Directions: The group of questions below consists of lettered choices followed by several numbered items. For each numbered item select the **one** lettered choice with which it is **most** closely associated. Each lettered choice may be used once, more than once, or not at all.

Questions 11–15

Match the pathogenetic factor with the disorder with which it is most closely associated.

(A) Waldenström's macroglobulinemia
(B) Poststreptococcal glomerulonephritis
(C) Hemolytic disease of the newborn
(D) Food allergy
(E) Contact dermatitis

11. $Rh_0(D)$ antigen
12. Excess monoclonal IgM
13. Antigen-reactive T cells
14. IgE antibody
15. Immune complexes

ANSWERS AND EXPLANATIONS

1. The answer is D. (*II D*) Immunotherapy for atopy involves the deliberate injection of the offending allergen, beginning at a low dosage and increasing to a maintenance dosage (i.e., the highest dose the patient can tolerate). The procedure stimulates production of IgG blocking antibody, which binds the allergen and forms complexes that are removed by the reticuloendothelial system, thus preventing the allergen from reaching and combining with the IgE on basophils and mast cells.

2. The answer is E. (*IV B 3*) Immune complex disorders manifest when antigen–antibody (immune) complexes—formed either locally or in the circulation—deposit in vascular or glomerular basement membrane and cause inflammation. The sequence of events that produces the immune complex reaction is as follows: The antigen–antibody complexes, once deposited, fix C1q, thus activating the classical complement pathway; as part of this reaction, C5a is generated, which is chemotactic for neutrophils; neutrophils then infiltrate the area and release lysosomal enzymes that destroy basement membrane.

3. The answer is A. (*V B*) Manifestation of delayed hypersensitivity requires intact, functioning T cells. Binding of antigen to specific antigen-reaction T cells causes the cells to release various soluble mediators, or lymphokines, which have various biological activities (e.g., macrophage migration inhibition factor, macrophage activation factor, macrophage chemotactic factor, and lymphotoxin).

4. The answer is D. (*II D 4 c*) One action of epinephrine is to stimulate adenyl cyclase, the enzyme responsible for converting adenosine triphosphate (ATP) to cyclic adenosine $3',5'$-monophosphate (cAMP). The latter blocks the release of mediators from mast cells and basophils. Theophylline, not epinephrine, inhibits phosphodiesterase, an enzyme that converts cAMP to AMP; thus, theophylline acts to preserve levels of cAMP essential for blocking mediator release. Epinephrine plays no significant role in inhibiting SRS-A, in inducing release of lymphokines, or in stimulating production of histamine.

5. The answer is C. (*VI E*) Amyloidosis is a disease characterized by deposition of amyloid fibrils in the vascular endothelium of various organs of the body. Two types of amyloidosis have been defined. Primary amyloidosis is a plasma cell dyscrasia characterized by the accumulation of amyloid fibrils that are composed primarily of immunoglobulin light chain fragments. This type of amyloidosis often is associated with multiple myeloma. Secondary amyloidosis refers to amyloidosis that occurs in the context of chronic infection or inflammation; the amyloid fibrils in secondary amyloidosis bear no structural resemblance to those seen in the primary form and have been termed "AA proteins."

6. The answer is E. (*VI A*) Multiple myeloma is one of several plasma cell dyscrasias—diseases that are characterized by the overproduction of immunoglobulins, or their fragments, by a single clone of plasma cells. Most cases of multiple myeloma involve plasma cell tumors of bone marrow that overproduce IgG.

7. The answer is E (all). (*II B 3*) Immediate hypersensitivity reactions (e.g., attacks of anaphylaxis, atopic allergy) are initiated by the interaction between antigens and cell-bound antibody—usually IgE. (Antigens that preferentially induce production of IgE are known as **allergens**.) Bridging of adjacent membrane-bound IgE molecules by allergen initiates degranulation and release of several pharmacologically active mediators from storage in mast cells and basophils. Among the various mediators are eosinophil chemotactic factor of anaphylaxis (ECF-A), histamine, bradykinin, platelet-activating factor (PAF), slow-reacting substance of anaphylaxis (SRS-A), serotonin, and prostaglandins.

8. The answer is B (1, 3). (*V B 3, D 1*) Delayed hypersensitivity (cell-mediated) tissue damage results from the interaction between sensitized T cells and specific antigen. This type of reaction occurs independent of antibody and complement but is dependent upon two types of T cells: T4+ cells and T8+ cells. Cortisone administration causes a decrease in blood lymphocytes, with a significantly greater reduction of T cells than B cells. Macrophage depletion also would inhibit cell-mediated reactions. Neither complement depletion nor antihistamine administration would be expected to affect cell-mediated reactions significantly.

9. The answer is C (2, 4). (*IV B*) The pathogenetic requirements for immune complex-induced glomerulonephritis include antigen (any of several antigens may be involved; they need not be derived from the kidney), antibody, complement, and neutrophils. The size of the immune complex is critical to its pathogenicity; complexes that are somewhat small, are not cleared from the circulation readily, and are deposited on blood vessel walls. Such immune complexes form in a region of antigen excess and are soluble, escape phagocytosis, penetrate the vascular endothelium, and lodge on the basement membrane. Activation of complement attracts neutrophils, which release lysosomal enzymes that destroy basement membrane. Recent studies have shown that, in humans, red blood cells participate in clearing immune complexes from the circulation; complexes that have been coated with C3b attach to C3b receptors on red blood cells, are transported to the liver and spleen, and then are removed from the red blood cells by phagocytes.

10. The answer is D (4). (*II A, B 2, C 2 b*) Allergic urticaria (hives) is one of the milder manifestations of immediate hypersensitivity—specifically, atopic allergy. A more serious, sometimes life-threatening form of immediate hypersensitivity is systemic anaphylaxis. Although other immunoglobulin classes have been implicated in immediate hypersensitivity reactions, the primary antibody responsible for such reactivity in humans is IgE.

11–15. The answers are: 11-C, 12-A, 13-E, 14-D, 15-B. [*II B 2; III C 1 b (1) (a); IV C 4; V C 1; VI B*] Hemolytic disease of the newborn occurs when an Rh-negative mother gives birth to an Rh-positive infant, the Rh antigen having been acquired from an Rh-positive father. The most commonly involved antigen is $Rh_0(D)$. For this condition to occur, the mother must be sensitized to blood group antigens of the infant's blood; sensitization usually occurs during a previous delivery. After sensitization, IgG antibodies to the acquired antigen are produced, which may cross the placenta and destroy fetal cells.

Waldenström's macroglobulinemia is a lymphocytic lymphoma characterized by overproduction of lymphocytes, plasma cells, and lymphocytes that resemble plasma cells. The most distinguishing feature of this disorder, however, is high levels of monoclonal IgM in the serum, which causes moderate to severe hyperviscosity of the blood. Plasmapheresis (plasma exchange) is used to treat the symptoms of the hyperviscosity syndrome (i.e., fatigue, confusion, increased bleeding tendency).

Delayed hypersensitivity (cell-mediated; type IV) reactions are T-cell–dependent reactions manifesting as inflammation at the site of antigen exposure. Tissue damage results from the interaction between sensitized T cells and specific antigen; antibody and complement are not required for these reactions. Contact dermatitis is a form of delayed hypersensitivity, which occurs in response to antigen exposure on skin. Delayed hypersensitivity reactions also occur in response to tumors as well as viral, bacterial, fungal, and parasitic infection.

Immediate hypersensitivity (type I) reactions are initiated by antigens reacting with cell-bound IgE antibody. The reaction may manifest in many ways, ranging from life-threatening systemic anaphylaxis to the lesser annoyance of atopic allergies, such as food allergies, allergic rhinitis (hay fever), and urticaria (hives).

Immune complex-mediated (type III) reactions are initiated by antigen–antibody complexes that form locally or in the circulation and deposit on vascular or glomerular basement membranes, where they cause inflammation. Glomerulonephritis is an example of systemic immune complex disease. This disease can occur in association with persistent infections or with the acute release of bacterial products, as in the case of poststreptococcal glomerulonephritis.

I. INTRODUCTION. A defect in the central mechanism underlying self-recognition (autotolerance, self-tolerance) can result in autoimmune responses, that is, immune responses of an individual to antigens present in the host's own tissue which can be mediated by humoral (circulating antibodies, immune complexes) or cellular (delayed hypersensitivity) mechanisms. Autoimmune diseases have been divided into two clinical types:

    A. Organ-specific (e.g., thyroiditis, pernicious anemia)

    B. Systemic [nonorgan-specific; e.g., systemic lupus erythematosus (SLE), rheumatoid arthritis]

II. ETIOLOGY

    A. Several theories have been proposed to explain autoimmune responses, or the termination of self-tolerance. It may represent an immunologic imbalance arising from the following:

        1. An excess of self-reactive helper T (Th)-cell activity induced, for example, by altered forms of self-antigen or with antigen that cross-reacts with self-antigen, which might be produced by a coupling of chemicals or drugs (e.g., hydralazine) or viruses to self-antigen: the modified chemical (drug)-host or viral-host antigens would then trigger a self-reactive Th-effect and elicit autoantibody production

        2. A bypass of the lack of requisite self-reactive Th-cell activity or bypass of the need for such Th-cell activity via polyclonal B-cell activation with materials such as bacterial lipopolysaccharide, Epstein-Barr virus, or purified protein derivative (PPD) of tuberculin

        3. A deficiency of suppressor T (Ts) cells designed to down-regulate the immune response to self-antigen

        4. Release of sequestered antigen (e.g., from lens of the eye, sperm) not ordinarily available for recognition by the immune system: release might occur via such means as trauma or infection

    B. Genetic predisposition

        1. There is clearly a role for genetic factors in autoimmune disease. The familial incidence that is seen is believed to be largely genetic rather than environmental and is thought to be associated with those genes [human leukocyte antigen (HLA)-DR] that code for the immune response to antigens. Most autoimmune diseases appear to be associated with DR2, DR3, DR4, and DR5. Some examples include rheumatoid arthritis, DR4; thyroiditis, DR5; multiple sclerosis, DR2; and SLE, DR3.

        2. Autoimmune diseases tend to occur at a higher frequency in females than in males (Table 10-1). For example, the incidence of SLE in women is six to nine times that in men, and rheumatoid arthritis is four times more common in females. The reason for this is still not certain, but it seems possible that sex hormones may play a role.

III. DIAGNOSIS

    A. General signs of autoimmune disease that may be of diagnostic importance include:

        1. Elevated serum gamma globulin levels

        2. Various autoantibodies

Table 10-1. Sex Ratio and Incidence of Certain Autoimmune Diseases

Disease	Female:Male	Estimated Incidence (USA)*
Rheumatoid arthritis	3:1	1000
Systemic lupus erythematosus	4:1	100
Multiple sclerosis	1:1	100
Sjögren's syndrome	9:1	0.5–1
Polymyositis–dermatomyositis	2:1	0.5–1
Ankylosing spondylitis	1:9	0.5–1

*Per 100,000

    3. Depressed levels of serum complement

    4. Immune complexes in serum

    5. Depressed levels of Ts cells

    6. Lesions detected on biopsy (e.g., glomerular lesions resulting from deposition of immune complexes)

  B. Diagnostic tests are designed to detect antibodies specific to the particular antigen involved in the disease. Certain facts should be pointed out, however.

    1. Autoantibodies are not unique to autoimmune disease; for example, antinuclear antibodies may be found in tuberculosis, histoplasmosis, malignant lymphoma, and other neoplasias.

    2. Patients with autoimmune disease may have more than one autoantibody.

    3. While SLE is associated with antinuclear antibodies and rheumatoid arthritis is associated with rheumatoid factor, both antibodies may be found in both diseases (Table 10-2).

IV. THERAPY for autoimmune disease involves several approaches. Agents such as nonsteroidal anti-inflammatory drugs (e.g., aspirin, indomethacin), steroidal anti-inflammatory drugs (e.g., cortisone, which may also be immunosuppressive), and immunosuppressive cytotoxic drugs (e.g., cyclophosphamide, azathioprine) are useful in treating disease symptoms. Anticholinesterase drugs and thymectomy are of value in myasthenia gravis. Plasmapheresis, or plasma exchange therapy, appears to be of value in certain diseases (e.g., Guillain-Barré, myasthenia gravis, Goodpasture's syndrome) by removing offending antibodies and immune complexes. In this technique, the plasma removed is replaced with normal serum albumin or fresh frozen plasma. Splenectomy is of value in hemolytic disease and idiopathic thrombocytopenic purpura.

V. REPRESENTATIVE AUTOIMMUNE DISEASES

  A. Acute disseminated encephalomyelitis may occur following vaccination (e.g., rabies immunization) or viral infection (e.g., measles, influenza).

    1. Clinicopathologic features

      a. Symptoms of encephalomyelitis include headache, backache, stiff neck, nausea, low-grade fever, malaise, weakness, or paralysis of extremities. Vaccination with attenuated viruses (e.g., measles, rubella) may produce symptoms such as elevated body temperature, convulsions, drowsiness that may progress to a comatose state, and paralysis of extremities, particularly the legs. Survivors of the acute stages of disease usually experience no permanent neurologic disorders, athough mental retardation, epileptic seizures, or even death can result.

      b. Pathologic examination reveals perivascular accumulation of macrophages, lymphocytes,

Table 10-2. Incidence of Antinuclear Antibodies and Rheumatoid Factor in Various Diseases

Diseases	Incidence	
	Antinuclear Antibodies	Rheumatoid Factor
Systemic lupus erythematosus	90% +	20%
Rheumatoid arthritis	20%	90% +
Sjögren's syndrome	70%	75%

and some neutrophils throughout the gray or white matter of the brain with variable demyelination.

2. **Immunologic findings** suggest that the disease represents a cell-mediated allergic response to basic protein of myelin similar to that seen in experimental allergic encephalomyelitis (see section V B). Antibodies to basic protein or myelin do not seem to be involved.

B. **Experimental allergic encephalomyelitis** is the experimental model for postvaccinal and postinfectious encephalomyelitis that can be induced in animals (e.g., guinea pig) by the injection of either homologous or heterologous brain or spinal cord extracts emulsified in complete Freund's adjuvant.

    1. **Clinicopathologic features**
       a. Within 2 to 3 weeks postsensitization, animals start to lose weight and then develop impaired righting reflex, ataxia, flaccid paralysis of the hind legs, urinary incontinence, and fecal impaction. Most animals ultimately die; however, some recover completely.
       b. Histologic lesions consist of perivascular inflammation (e.g., lymphocytes, mononuclear cells, plasma cells) throughout the brain and spinal cord and demyelination of nerve tissue.

    2. **Immunologic findings**
       a. The encephalitogenic factor appears to be certain polypeptide sequences of myelin basic protein. Animals demonstrate classic cutaneous delayed hypersensitivity to basic protein, and the disease can be passively transferred with lymphoid cells.
       b. Although both B cells and T cells respond to basic protein, the T cell appears to be responsible for the disease (demyelination). Antibodies to basic protein are formed but they correlate poorly with disease and are unable to passively transfer disease.

C. **Chronic thyroiditis (Hashimoto's thyroiditis)** is a disease of the thyroid that mainly affects women in the age group between 30 and 50 years.

    1. **Clinicopathologic features**
       a. **The thyroid gland may be enlarged** (goiter) and firm or hard. Histologic examination reveals a lymphocyte and plasma cell infiltrate, disappearance of colloid, and varying amounts of fibrosis.
       b. As the disease progresses, signs of diminished thyroid function (**hypothyroidism**) may be seen, for example, in low values of circulating thyroid hormones and decreased thyroidal radioiodine uptake.

    2. **Immunologic findings**
       a. Various antibodies to thyroid-specific antigens can be demonstrated.
          (1) Antibody to **thyroglobulin** will precipitate thyroglobulin and also agglutinate tanned red blood cells coated with thyroglobulin (passive hemagglutination). It may also be detected via radioimmunoassay, immunofluorescence, and enzyme-linked immunosorbent assay (ELISA) [see Chapter 8].
          (2) Antibody to thyroid microsomal antigen can be detected by complement fixation and hemagglutination tests (see Chapter 8).
          (3) Antibody to a second colloid antigen has been detected but is not well characterized.
       b. Experimental animals (e.g., rabbit, guinea pig, rat, mouse) injected with homologous or autologous thyroid extract incorporated in complete Freund's adjuvant develop lesions and other features similar to those seen in human disease. Delayed hypersensitivity reaction to thyroid extract can also be demonstrated.
       c. The relative importance of T cells and B cells in the pathogenesis of disease is not yet clearly resolved. Both cell types may be essential for maximum effect. Antibody-dependent cellular cytotoxic (ADCC) reaction may also be involved.

D. **Multiple sclerosis** is a relapsing disease with exacerbations between periods of remission. Epidemiologic studies have revealed high-risk and low-risk areas of the world and a possible role for a transmissible agent. Evidence that susceptibility may be genetically determined is suggested by a close association with HLA-DR2.

    1. **Clinicopathologic features**
       a. Symptoms include motor weakness, ataxia, impaired vision, urinary bladder dysfunction, paresthesias, and mental aberrations.
       b. Inflammatory lesions (**sclerotic plaques**) are confined to the myelin in the central nervous system and consist of mononuclear cell infiltrates and demyelination.

    2. **Immunologic findings**
       a. The cause of multiple sclerosis remains unknown, but **the clustering character of cases**

suggests an infectious agent. Of interest in this regard is the finding that patients tend to have elevated levels of antibodies to measles virus in their serum and spinal fluid; however, the exact role of measles virus is unknown. There is, in fact, evidence that other viral agents may also be involved.

  b. **Increased concentrations of IgG in the spinal fluid** are seen in most patients. The ratio of spinal fluid-to-serum immunoglobulin is reduced, and there is evidence that local IgG synthesis occurs in nerve tissue based on the oligoclonal pattern seen on electrophoresis.

  c. Patients tend to show **suppressed levels of circulating T cells** and **increased levels of B cells**. This may explain the decreased delayed hypersensitivity response to measles seen in patients.

E. Graves' disease (thyrotoxicosis, hyperthyroidism) results from the overproduction of thyroid hormone (thyroxine).

  1. Clinicopathologic features. Patients demonstrate fatigue, nervousness, increased sweating, palpitations, weight loss, and heat intolerance.

  2. Immunologic findings
  a. An increase in the number of peripheral B cells correlates with the severity of the disease.
  b. Patients also show a decrease in the percentage of T cells in blood, mainly Ts cells.
  c. Current evidence suggests that patients produce antibodies to thyrotropin receptors, which are referred to as **thyroid-stimulating antibodies** since they compete with thyroid stimulating hormone (thyrotropin, which is made in the pituitary) for receptor sites on the thyroid cell membrane and mimic the action of thyrotropin. The end result is overproduction of thyroid hormone and hyperthyroidism.
  d. Since the antibodies to thyrotropin receptors are IgG, they can cross the placenta and cause hyperthyroidism in newborns of diseased mothers. The condition resolves spontaneously when the maternal IgG is catabolized by the infant over a period of several weeks.
  e. In several studies of HLA antigen frequencies in patients, increased frequencies of HLA-B8 and HLA-D3 have been found.

F. Guillain-Barré syndrome (acute idiopathic polyneuritis) commonly occurs after an infectious disease (e.g., measles, hepatitis) or after vaccination (e.g., influenza) and affects all age groups.

  1. Clinicopathologic features
  a. Symptoms include progressive weakness, first of the lower extremities, and then of upper extremities and respiratory muscles, and paralysis. Most patients recover normal function in 6 to 10 months.
  b. Examination of peripheral nerve tissue reveals a perivascular mononuclear cell infitrate and demyelination.

  2. Immunologic findings
  a. A similar disease can be produced in experimental animals by injection of peripheral nerve extracts, or peptides derived therefrom, incorporated in complete Freund's adjuvant. **The experimental disease appears to be cell-mediated** as evidenced by sensitivity of lymphocytes to nerve extracts, release of lymphokines from sensitized lymphocytes, and passive transfer of disease with sensitized cells. Antinerve antibodies can be detected but seem to play no role in pathogenesis.
  b. The human disease has several of the same immunologic features as the experimental animal model (e.g., lymphocytes sensitive to peripheral nerve extracts, lymphokine production, and antinerve antibodies).

G. Myasthenia gravis is a chronic disease resulting from faulty neuromuscular transmission.

  1. Clinicopathologic features
  a. The disease is characterized by muscle weakness and fatigability involving particularly ocular, pharyngeal, facial, laryngeal, and skeletal muscles.
  b. Muscle weakness and neuromuscular dysfunction result from **depletion of acetylcholine receptors at the myoneural junction**.

  2. Immunologic findings
  a. About 60% to 80% of patients have an enlarged thymus, and 80% to 90% of patients have antibodies (frequently an IgG3 isotype) against the acetylcholine receptor. It is this antibody that apparently binds to acetylcholine receptors at the myoneural junction, causing endocytosis of the receptors.
  b. Injection of experimental animals with purified acetylcholine receptor incorporated in complete Freund's adjuvant induces **experimental myasthenia gravis** that closely mimics human disease. Serum from animals with experimentally induced disease, as well as from human patients, will passively transfer the syndrome to normal animals.

    c. Although there is evidence that cellular immunity may also be involved (e.g., lymphocyte stimulation by purified acetylcholine receptor and passive transfer with lymphoid cells), it would appear that the antibody response is more intimately involved.

    d. Complement-binding immune complexes may cause further problems at the myoneural junction.

H. Systemic lupus erythematosus is a chronic, multiorgan disorder that predominantly affects young women of childbearing age.

  1. Clinicopathologic features

    a. General symptoms include **malaise, fever, lethargy,** and **weight loss.**

    b. Multiple tissues that are involved include the skin, mucosa, blood vessels, kidney, brain, and blood.

      (1) The most characteristic feature is the **butterfly rash**, an erythematous rash that occurs over the nose and cheeks. Other lesions (e.g., discoid, psoriasiform) or eruptions (e.g., maculopapular, bullous) have also been described.

      (2) Renal involvement occurs in 50% of patients with SLE. **Diffuse proliferative glomerulonephritis** and **membranous glomerulonephritis** are common manifestations. Death usually results from renal failure or infection.

      (3) Central nervous system (CNS) manifestations appear in 50% of patients and include depression, psychoses, seizures, and sensorimotor neuropathies.

  2. Immunologic findings

    a. The discovery of the **lupus erythematosus (LE) cell phenomenon** led to the current understanding of the immunologic basis of SLE. When peripheral blood from a patient is incubated at 37°C for 30 to 60 minutes, the lymphocytes swell and extrude their nuclear material. This material, through opsonization by anti-DNA antibody and complement, is phagocytized by neutrophils, which are now called LE cells.

    b. The detection of **antinuclear antibodies** via the indirect immunofluorescence technique (see Chapter 8) is of diagnostic importance in SLE (see Table 10-2). Three primary types of antibodies to DNA (**either IgG or IgM**) can be detected:

      (1) Antibodies to single-stranded DNA (ss-DNA)

      (2) Antibodies to double-stranded DNA (ds-DNA). Antibodies to ds-DNA (complement-fixing) are most closely associated with active SLE and the renal disease (glomerulonephritis) that is triggered by deposition of immune complexes (DNA–antibody–complement) on the basement membrane of blood vessels of renal glomeruli (see Chapter 9).

      (3) Antibodies that react with both ss-DNA and ds-DNA

    c. In some patients, in addition to anti-DNA antibodies, antibodies are formed against RNA, erythrocytes, platelets, mitochondria, ribosomes, lysosomes, thromboplastin, and thrombin. Some patients demonstrate a positive test for rheumatoid factor (see section V I 2 a and Chapter 8).

    d. Most patients show **hypergammaglobulinemia** and **reduced serum complement levels** (particularly C3 and C4) due to increased utilization caused by immune complex formation.

    e. There is a drop in the number of T cells and a subsequent impaired ability to develop delayed hypersensitivity. Antibodies cytotoxic for T cells correlate with this T-cell deficiency.

    f. Mice of the NZB/NZW strain spontaneously develop disease with essentially all of the features of SLE (e.g., LE cells, antinuclear antibodies, immune complex glomerulonephritis, T-cell deficiency). In mice there is a deficiency of Ts cells that would normally be expected to suppress autoantibody formation.

I. Rheumatoid arthritis is a chronic inflammatory joint disease, with possible systemic involvement as well.

  1. Clinicopathologic features

    a. General symptoms include weight loss, malaise, fever, fatigue, and weakness. The disease affects primarily females and is associated with HLA-DR4, which may impart genetic susceptibility.

    b. An unknown etiologic agent initiates a nonspecific immune response. An inflammatory joint lesion that begins in the synovial membrane can become proliferative, destroying adjacent cartilage and bone and resulting in joint deformity.

    c. Serum protein electrophoresis may show hypergammaglobulinemia and hypoalbuminemia.

  2. Immunologic findings

    a. Rheumatoid factor. A hallmark of rheumatoid arthritis is the presence of rheumatoid factor, an immunoglobulin (mainly IgM but also IgG and IgA) produced by the B cells and plasma cells in the synovial membrane with **antibody specificity for the Fc fragment of IgG.**

    (1) IgG is apparently altered in some way to appear as "nonself," perhaps by binding to another antigen. IgM and IgG rheumatoid factors are the primary contributors to immunoglobulin production of the rheumatoid synovial membrane.

    (2) Rheumatoid factor is present in the serum of most (possibly 80% to 90%+) patients with established rheumatoid arthritis, and these patients generally have more severe disease than patients without rheumatoid factor (see Table 10-2).

  b. The **joint synovial fluid contains immune complexes** consisting of **rheumatoid factor–IgG–complement.** Rheumatoid factor can trigger an immune response in two ways.

    (1) Immune complex activation of complement. Rheumatoid factor may combine with IgG away from its antibody combining site, leaving the IgG molecule free to combine with other antibodies and form larger "poly-IgG complexes." These aggregates can reach a size large enough to fix complement and activate complement pathways (both classic and alternate pathways) with production of neutrophil chemotactic factors (C5a, C5b67).

    (2) Immune complex ingestion. An inflammatory response is amplified as aggregates of IgG rheumatoid factor are phagocytized by macrophages (which release lymphokines) and neutrophils (which release digestive enzymes). Neutrophils that have engulfed immune complexes are called **rheumatoid arthritis (RA) cells.** Compared to serum levels of IgG, synovial levels of IgG (but not IgM) rheumatoid factor are relatively reduced, suggesting that phagocytosis of IgG rheumatoid factor may have a specific role in the inflammatory response.

  c. Many patients with rheumatoid arthritis also have antinuclear antibodies (see Table 10-2).

J. Sjögren's syndrome, also called **sicca syndrome**, is a chronic inflammatory disease that affects multiple systems of the body, although the primary target appears to be secretory glands such as the lacrimal and salivary glands.

  1. Clinicopathologic features

    a. The disease is characterized by dry eyes (**keratoconjunctivitis sicca**) and dry mouth (**xerostomia**), usually with an associated connective tissue disease such as rheumatoid arthritis or SLE.

    b. Dryness of the nose, larynx, and respiratory tract is also seen. In females, where the disease is most often seen, the vaginal mucosa is also dry.

  2. Immunologic findings

    a. Patients demonstrate **hypergammaglobulinemia**, suggesting excessive B-cell activity, and several types of autoantibodies, such as rheumatoid factor, antinuclear antibodies, and antibody to salivary duct epithelium (see Table 10-2).

    b. Salivary and lacrimal glands are infiltrated with plasma cells, B cells, and T cells. Some patients show a quantitative and qualitative T-cell suppression in peripheral blood. All of these features suggest an immunologic etiology.

K. Hemolytic diseases that have been characterized as having an **autoimmune** basis include warm antibody hemolytic anemia, cold antibody hemolytic anemia, and paroxysmal cold hemoglobinuria (see Chapter 9 for discussion of other forms of immunologically mediated anemias).

  1. Clinicopathologic features. Classic symptoms include fatigue, fever, jaundice, and splenomegaly referable to the presence of antibodies directed against "self" red blood cell antigens and the resultant anemia.

  2. Immunologic findings

    a. Warm antibody hemolytic anemia

      (1) This is the most common type of autoimmune hemolytic disease, involving so-called warm antibodies, which show optimum reactivity at 37°C. They are primarily IgG, are poor at complement fixing, and can be detected on the red blood cell surface by the antiglobulin (Coombs) test.

      (2) Using appropriate techniques, various patterns of red blood cell coating can be detected in different patients. Cells can be coated with IgG alone, IgG plus complement, or complement alone.

      (3) The warm antibody is directed primarily against Rh determinants, and antibody-coated red cells appear to be opsonized for phagocytosis primarily in the spleen.

    b. Cold antibody hemolytic anemia

      (1) Cold antibodies show optimum reactivity at 4°C. They are primarily of the IgM class, fix complement, and agglutinate red blood cells directly, without the requirement for Coombs antiglobulin.

      (2) The specificity of the IgM is anti-I or anti-i.

      (3) Cold agglutinins may also be detected secondary to infections (e.g., mycoplasmal pneumonia).

   c. Paroxysmal cold hemoglobinuria is a rare syndrome associated with a cold antibody (Donath-Landsteiner) of the IgG class directed against red blood cell antigen P.

      (1) The antibody is biphasic in that it sensitizes cells in the cold, usually below 15°C, and then hemolyzes them when the temperature is elevated to 37°C.

      (2) Patients demonstrate symptoms (e.g., fever, pain in extremities, jaundice, hemoglobinuria) following exposure to cold.

L. Idiopathic thrombocytopenic purpura, which may be either acute or chronic, results from antibody-mediated platelet destruction. In children, it is sometimes preceded by a viral infection.

   1. Clinicopathologic features. Patients demonstrate petechiae and various bleeding problems in their gums, gastrointestinal tract, and genitourinary tract. The peripheral blood platelet counts are profoundly suppressed (i.e., less than 100,000/μl), as is platelet survival time.

   2. Immunologic findings

      a. IgG antibodies specific for platelets can be demonstrated. Antibody-coated platelets are sequestered and destroyed by macrophages of the spleen primarily, and the liver. Since the simple, more routine laboratory techniques are not sensitive enough to detect antibodies, more sophisticated tests must be used (e.g., enzyme-linked immunosorbent assay or radiolabeled Coombs antiglobulin test).

      b. Idiopathic thrombocytopenic purpura may sometimes be drug-induced via such drugs as sulfonamides, antihistamines, quinidine, and quinine. In these instances, the problem is caused by adsorption of drug–antibody complexes onto the platelet surface and subsequent complement activation. Treatment consists of withholding the drug.

M. Goodpasture's syndrome is a rare, progressive disease of the lungs and kidneys. The disease occurs in all age groups, affecting mainly young men. The prognosis is poor.

   1. Clinicopathologic features

      a. Classic symptoms include pulmonary hemorrhage, hemoptysis, hematuria, and glomerulonephritis. Pulmonary infiltrates may show on x-rays.

      b. Immunofluorescence examination reveals linear deposits of immunoglobulin (usually IgG) and complement on alveolar and glomerular basement membranes.

   2. Immunologic findings

      a. IgG appears to represent an antibody specific for an antigen shared by kidney and lung basement membranes.

      b. Some cases have characteristics suggestive of an immune complex phenomenon.

N. Pernicious anemia results from defective red blood cell maturation due to faulty absorption of vitamin B_{12}. Normally, dietary B_{12} is transported across the small intestine into the body as a complex with intrinsic factor synthesized by parietal cells in gastric mucosa. In patients with pernicious anemia, the process is blocked.

   1. Clinicopathologic features

      a. The hallmark of the disease is the progressive destruction of stomach glands associated with loss of parietal cells which secrete intrinsic factor. This leads to failure of B_{12} absorption.

      b. The gastric mucosa is infiltrated with mononuclear leukocytes and neutrophils.

      c. Defective red blood cell maturation leads to weakness, loss of appetite, fatigability, pallor, and weight loss.

   2. Immunologic findings

      a. Patients produce antibodies (mainly IgG) to three different gastric parietal cell antigens, all of which are cell-specific. In addition, antibody to intrinsic factor is produced.

      b. Antibody to intrinsic factor may either block attachment of B_{12} to intrinsic factor or bind to intrinsic factor or to the intrinsic factor–B_{12} complex.

      c. In some patients, cell-mediated immunity to intrinsic factor and parietal cell antigen has also been detected.

O. Bullous (vesicular) diseases are chronic dermatologic problems that result when destruction of intercellular bridges (desmosomes) interferes with cohesion of the epidermis, leading to the formation of blisters.

1. Clinicopathologic features
   a. Pemphigus vulgaris is an erosive disease of the skin and mucous membranes, with intra-epidermal blisters.
   b. Bullous pemphigoid is a bullous disease, primarily of the skin, usually seen in middle-aged and older persons. The blisters form beneath the epidermis at the dermal–epidermal junction.

2. Immunologic findings
   a. Pemphigus vulgaris skin lesions, when examined by immunofluorescence, show deposition of antibody (mainly IgG) and complement components in squamous intercellular spaces.
   b. Bullous pemphigoid lesions, by immunofluorescence examination, demonstrate deposition of antibody and complement along skin basement membrane. Circulating antibasement membrane antibodies can also be detected.

P. Polymyositis–dermatomyositis is an acute or chronic inflammatory disease of the muscle and skin.

1. Clinicopathologic features. Patients demonstrate weakness of striated muscle, with some muscle pain and tenderness, plus a characteristic skin rash.

2. Immunologic findings
   a. Hypergammaglobulinemia is common, along with deposition of immunoglobulin and complement in the vessel walls of the skin and muscle.
   b. Cellular immunity may also play a role in pathogenesis as judged from studies of cellular passive transfer and lymphokine release from lymphocytes.

STUDY QUESTIONS

Directions: Each question below contains five suggested answers. Choose the **one best** response to each question.

1. All of the following signs are of diagnostic importance in autoimmune disease EXCEPT

(A) lesions detected on biopsy
(B) immune complexes in serum
(C) depressed levels of serum complement
(D) depressed levels of suppressor T (Ts) cells
(E) depressed serum gamma globulin levels

2. The Donath-Landsteiner antibody is characteristic of

(A) warm antibody hemolytic anemia
(B) cold antibody hemolytic anemia
(C) paroxysmal cold hemoglobinuria
(D) idiopathic thrombocytopenic purpura
(E) pernicious anemia

Directions: Each question below contains four suggested answers of which **one or more** is correct. Choose the answer

A if **1, 2, and 3** are correct
B if **1 and 3** are correct
C if **2 and 4** are correct
D if **4** is correct
E if **1, 2, 3, and 4** are correct

3. Antinuclear antibodies and rheumatoid factor are commonly associated with

(1) rheumatoid arthritis
(2) Sjögren's syndrome
(3) systemic lupus erythematosus
(4) idiopathic thrombocytopenic purpura

4. Organ-specific autoimmune diseases include

(1) thyroiditis
(2) systemic lupus erythematosus
(3) pernicious anemia
(4) rheumatoid arthritis

5. Immunofluorescence examination of tissue from patients with Goodpasture's syndrome reveals linear deposits of immunoglobulin and complement on

(1) stratified squamous epithelium
(2) alveolar basement membrane
(3) skin basement membrane
(4) glomerular basement membrane

6. Termination of self-tolerance and resultant autoimmune disease could theoretically be triggered by the

(1) excess of self-reactive helper T (Th) cells
(2) bypass of the need for self-reactive Th-cell activity
(3) deficiency of suppressor T (Ts) cells
(4) release of sequestered self-antigen

7. A T-cell response to basic protein of myelin appears to be responsible for the pathogenesis of

(1) experimental allergic encephalomyelitis
(2) Grave's disease
(3) acute disseminated encephalomyelitis
(4) Hashimoto's thyroiditis

8. The chronic inflammation characteristic of Sjögren's syndrome affects multiple body systems, including primarily the

(1) gastric glands
(2) lacrimal glands
(3) thyroid gland
(4) salivary glands

SUMMARY OF DIRECTIONS

A	B	C	D	E
1, 2, 3 only	1, 3 only	2, 4 only	4 only	All are correct

at 1→8°C

9. The warm antibody involved in autoimmune hemolytic disease

(1) requires Coombs antiglobulin for detection
A (2) primarily consists of IgG
(3) fixes complement poorly
(4) demonstrates specificity for the P red blood cell antigen

lupus - 85% in ♀
↳ C2 deficiency

10. Autoimmune diseases can be characterized by

↗ and ↗ Estrogen

(1) a tendency to occur more frequently in women
(2) treatment with nonsteroidal anti-inflammatory agents   *Aspirin*
(3) familial incidence   *& indomethacin*
E (4) autoantibodies in the serum

Directions: The group of questions below consists of lettered choices followed by several numbered items. For each numbered item select the **one** lettered choice with which it is **most** closely associated. Each lettered choice may be used once, more than once, or not at all.

Questions 11–15

For each immunologic characteristic, select the disease most closely associated with it.

(A) Systemic lupus erythematosus (SLE)
(B) Pernicious anemia
(C) Myasthenia gravis
(D) Multiple sclerosis
(E) Rheumatoid arthritis

B 11. Antibodies to gastric parietal cell antigens and to intrinsic factor

E 12. Immunoglobulins with a specificity for the Fc fragment of IgG

C 13. Antibodies to acetylcholine receptor

A 14. Glomerulonephritis triggered by deposition of DNA–antibody–complement complexes on blood vessel basement membrane

D 15. Elevated levels of antibodies to measles virus in serum and spinal fluid

ANSWERS AND EXPLANATIONS

1. The answer is E. (*III A 1, 3–6*) Elevated, not depressed, serum gamma globulin levels are one of several general signs of autoimmune disease that may be of diagnostic importance. Other signs include depressed levels of serum complement or suppressor T (Ts) cells, lesions detected on biopsy, and the presence of immune complexes in the serum.

2. The answer is C. (*V K 2*) Cold antibody hemolytic anemia involves antibody optimally reactive in the IgM class. Paroxysmal cold hemoglobinuria is a rare type of autoimmune hemolytic disease that is associated with the Donath-Landsteiner antibody, a cold antibody of the IgG class directed against red blood cell antigen P. Warm antibody hemolytic anemia involves primarily IgG antibodies; the antibodies are considered to be "warm" due to their optimum reactivity at 37°C. Idiopathic thrombocytopenic purpura results from antibody-mediated platelet destruction. Pernicious anemia results from defective red blood cell maturation due to immunologically mediated faulty absorption of vitamin B_{12}.

3. The answer is A (1, 2, 3). [*V H 2 b, c, I 2 b (2), d, J 2 a; Table 10-2*] While systemic lupus erythematosus (SLE) is associated with antinuclear antibodies and rheumatoid arthritis is associated with rheumatoid factor, both antibodies may be found in both diseases as well as in Sjögren's syndrome. In idiopathic thrombocytopenic purpura, IgG antibodies specific for platelets cause the cells to be destroyed by macrophages of the spleen and liver.

4. The answer is B (1, 3). (*I A, B*) Autoimmune diseases tend to represent a spectrum in which the immune response is directed against just one organ in the body (organ-specific), as in Hashimoto's thyroiditis (target = thyroid) and pernicious anemia (target = gastric tissue), as well as against antigens widespread throughout the body (systemic), as in systemic lupus erythematosus [SLE] (target = cell nuclear material) and rheumatoid arthritis (target = IgG). In the case of organ-specific disease, the lesions are generally restricted because the antigen in that organ is the target of the immunologic attack. In systemic autoimmune disease, antigen–antibody complex deposition in, for example, the kidneys or joints, is involved, which explains the more disseminated features of the disease.

5. The answer is C (2, 4). (*V M 2 a*) In Goodpasture's syndrome, symptoms referable to both the lungs (pulmonary hemorrhage, hemoptysis) and kidneys (glomerulonephritis, hematuria) are seen. The deposits of immunoglobulin (usually IgG) on alveolar and glomerular basement membranes represent antibody specific for antigen shared by the kidneys and lungs. The prognosis for patients is poor.

6. The answer is E (all). (*II A 1–4*) All of the theories listed have found some support. An excess of self-reactive helper T (Th) cell activity may be produced by altered forms of self-antigen triggered by virus (e.g., influenza) coupling to the self-antigen (acute disseminated encephalomyelitis). There is convincing evidence that certain polyclonal B-cell activators (e.g., bacterial lipopolysaccharide) may precipitate autoantibody production by bypassing the need for self-reactive Th-cell activity. If a population of suppressor T (Ts) cells is involved in down-regulating the immune response to self, then a deficiency of such cells may terminate self-tolerance. In mice of the NZB/NZW strain that spontaneously develop a disease like systemic lupus erythematosus (SLE), there is a deficiency of Ts cells. Autoantibody production following release of sequestered antigen has also been demonstrated (e.g., autoantibody formation against sperm after vasectomy).

7. The answer is B (1, 3). (*V A, B*). In acute disseminated encephalomyelitis in humans and in the animal experimental model, there is perivascular accumulation of lymphocytes and other cells throughout nervous tissue along with variable demyelination. The latter appears to be triggered via a T-cell–mediated response to basic protein of myelin.

8. The answer is C (2, 4). (*V J 1 a, b*) Sjögren's syndrome is characterized by dry eyes (keratoconjunctivitis sicca) and dry mouth (xerostomia). Salivary and lacrimal glands are infiltrated with plasma cells, B cells and T cells, suggesting an immunologic etiology. Patients also demonstrate hypergammaglobulinemia and several types of autoantibodies such as rheumatoid factor, antinuclear antibodies, and antibody to salivary duct epithelium.

9. The answer is A (1, 2, 3). [*V K 2 a (1), (3)*] The most common type of autoimmune hemolytic disease involves so-called warm antibodies which show optimum reactivity at 37°C, are primarily IgG, are poor at complement fixation, and can be detected by the antiglobulin (Coombs) test. The antibody is directed primarily against Rh antigens on the red blood cells.

10. The answer is E (all). (*II B; III B; IV*) Most autoimmune diseases are more common in females (e.g., approximately 85% of patients with systemic lupus erythematosus (SLE) are women). This implies that sex hormones may play a precipitating (estrogens) or controlling (androgens) role. Certain diseases have increased incidence in association with particular HLA antigens, most particularly antigens coded for in the D/DR locus. Aspirin and indomethacin are commonly used to control certain symptoms of autoimmune disease. Most diagnostic tests rely on examination of serum for decreased complement levels or suppressor T (Ts) cells or increases in immune complexes and gamma globulin.

11–15. The answers are: 11-B, 12-E, 13-C, 14-A, 15-D. [*V D 2 a, G 1 b, H 2 b (2), I 2 a, N 2 a*] Pernicious anemia results from defective red blood cell maturation due to faulty absorption of vitamin B_{12}. Normally, dietary B_{12} is transported across the small intestine as a complex with intrinsic factor synthesized by parietal cells in gastric mucosa. In this disease, the process is blocked due to the presence of antibodies to parietal cells and to intrinsic factor.

Rheumatoid arthritis is a chronic inflammatory joint disease; joint deformity is common. A hallmark of the disease is the presence, in serum and synovial fluid, of rheumatoid factors which are antibodies (mainly IgM) with a specificity for the Fc fragment of IgG. Rheumatoid factor–IgG–complement in joint fluid attracts neutrophil complexes which damage synovium by discharging their lysosomal contents.

Myasthenia gravis results from faulty neuromuscular transmission triggered by depletion of acetylcholine receptors at the myoneural junction. Autoantibody binds to acetylcholine receptors at the myoneural junction, causing the endocytosis of receptors. Complement-binding immune complexes may cause further problems at the junction.

Systemic lupus erythematosus (SLE) is a chronic, systemic, multiorgan disease characterized by the production of a variety of autoantibodies versus, for example, DNA, RNA, erythrocytes, platelets, and ribosomes. However, anti-DNA antibodies are most closely associated with active disease and the glomerulonephritis triggered by deposition of DNA–antibody–complement complexes on the basement membrane of blood vessels of renal glomeruli.

Multiple sclerosis is a relapsing neurologic disorder associated with lesions (plaques) confined to the central nervous system consisting of mononuclear cell infiltrates and demyelination. The cause is unknown but patients tend to have elevated levels, in serum and spinal fluid, of antibodies to measles virus. The exact role of measles virus is unknown. Other viral agents may also be involved.

11
Immunodeficiency Disorders

I. INTRODUCTION. In view of the complex nature of the immune response, it is not surprising that a wide array of deficiencies exist, heralded primarily by recurrent infection, chronic infection, unusual (opportunistic) infecting agents, and a poor response to treatment. Occasionally other manifestations such as skin rash, hepatosplenomegaly, diarrhea, and evidence of autoimmunity are symptoms of compromised host defenses. When an immunodeficiency syndrome is suspected in a given individual based on the presence of persistent and recurrent infections, the workup of the patient includes a number of valuable assessment procedures (see Chapter 8 section IV).

In this chapter, immunodeficiency is discussed under six categories: phagocytic cell defects; B-cell deficiency; T-cell deficiency; combined B-cell and T-cell deficiency; secondary immunodeficiency; and complement deficiency.

II. PHAGOCYTIC CELL DEFECTS

A. **Quantitative defects.** Although defects can occur in most phagocytic cells, emphasis is given here to neutrophils. In **quantitative defects in polymorphonuclear leukocytes (neutrophils)**, referred to as **neutropenia or granulocytopenia**, the total number of normal, circulating cells is suppressed.

1. Their numbers can drop through decreased production, which is associated with several causes, including:
   a. Administration of certain bone marrow depressant drugs (e.g., nitrogen mustard)
   b. Leukemia
   c. Inherited conditions, such as reticular dysgenesis (de Vaal syndrome), where there appears to be defective development of all bone marrow stem cells, including myeloid precursors

2. Circulating neutrophils are also suppressed through increased destruction, which is associated with conditions including:
   a. Autoimmune phenomena versus neutrophil antigens. Neutropenia has been associated with spontaneously arising autoantibody that inhibits granulopoiesis. It has also been seen following the administration of certain drugs (e.g., quinidine and oxacillin) which may induce antibodies capable of opsonizing normal neutrophils.
   b. Hypersplenism characterized by exaggeration of the destructive functions of the spleen, and resultant deficiency of peripheral blood elements.

B. **Qualitative defects.** In qualitative disorders, the phagocytic cells fail to engulf and kill microorganisms. The defect may reside in chemotaxis, ingestion, and killing and digestion, or all three.

1. **Chronic granulomatous disease** is characterized by recurrent infections with various gram-negative (e.g., *Escherichia*, *Serratia*, and *Klebsiella*) and gram-positive (e.g., *Staphylococcus*) microorganisms. It is primarily an X-linked recessive disorder, and onset is in the first 2 years of life.
   a. **Clinical features**
      (1) Associated findings often include hepatosplenomegaly, lymphadenopathy, draining lymph nodes, and pneumonia.
      (2) **Granuloma formation** occurs in many organs, and it appears to reflect the inability of, first, neutrophils and then tissue macrophages to kill ingested microorganisms. The neutrophils fail to respond to phagocytosis with the reaction of normal neutrophils, which involves increases in oxygen consumption activity of the pentose phosphate

pathway (hexose monophosphate shunt) and hydrogen peroxide production. This apparently is due to reduction in intracellular reduced nicotinamide adenine dinucleotide (NADH) or reduced nicotinamide adenine dinucleotide phosphate (NADPH). There is also decreased iodination and superoxide anion production and absence of cytochrome b. The result is **suppression of intracellular killing of ingested microorganisms**.

 b. The **diagnosis** is dependent on demonstration in vitro of defective killing by neutrophils. B-cell and T-cell function and complement levels are generally normal.

 c. Treatment involves the use of antibiotics appropriate for the infectious agent and, possibly, temporary maintenance with neutrophil infusions from a family member.

2. Myeloperoxidase deficiency is seen in some patients with recurrent microbial infections. Myeloperoxidase is an important microbicidal agent contained in normal neutrophils. Hydrogen peroxide is formed in these patients in normal amounts; however, both myeloperoxide and hydrogen peroxide are necessary for neutrophil killing function.

3. Chédiak-Higashi syndrome is a relatively rare disease of humans and of a variety of animals (e.g., mink, cattle, and mice).

 a. Clinical features. This syndrome is characterized by partial albinism and recurrent, severe pyogenic infections with primarily streptococci and staphylococci. The patient's neutrophils contain abnormal, giant lysosomes, which can apparently fuse with the phagosome but which are impaired in their ability to release their contents, resulting in a delayed killing of ingested microorganisms.

 b. Diagnosis. There is abnormal neutrophil production, chemotaxis, and microtubule function and depressed lysosomal enzyme levels in the face of apparently normal NAD, B-cell, T-cell, and complement function.

 c. Treatment involves the use of antibiotics appropriate for the type of infection.

 d. Prognosis is poor. Most patients die in childhood.

4. Job's syndrome [hyperimmunoglobulinemia E (hyper-IgE) syndrome]

 a. Clinical features. Job's syndrome is characterized by recurrent "cold" (i.e., lacking the normal inflammatory response) staphylococcal abscesses, chronic eczema, and otitis media.

 b. Diagnosis

  (1) Neutrophils demonstrate normal ingestion and killing activity but defective chemotaxis.

  (2) Serum levels of IgE are extremely high in association with increased specificity for staphylococcal antigens.

  (3) Eosinophilia may be present, and the number of suppressor T (Ts) cells may be reduced.

 c. Treatment involves the use of antibiotics appropriate for the infectious agent.

5. Lazy leukocyte syndrome is characterized by susceptibility to severe microbial infections, neutropenia, defective chemotactic response by neutrophils, and an abnormal inflammatory response. **Treatment** involves antibiotics appropriate for the infectious agent.

III. B-CELL DEFICIENCY DISORDERS

A. Bruton's X-linked hypogammaglobulinemia manifests as recurrent infections (e.g., sinusitis, pneumonia, and meningitis) that are caused by organisms such as *Streptococcus*, *Haemophilus*, *Staphylococcus*, and *Pseudomonas* beginning when the infant is 5 to 9 months of age. The primary bacterial infections do not induce immunoglobulin synthesis. Cellular immunity is normal in these patients.

 1. Immunologic findings include:

  a. Low serum levels of all classes of immunoglobulins

  b. Lack of circulating B cells

  c. Lack of germinal centers and plasma cells in lymph nodes

  d. Absent or hypoplastic tonsils and Peyer's patches

  e. Intact T-cell function

 2. Treatment consists of intramuscular or intravenous injections of commercial pooled human gamma globulin, usually administered monthly. Fresh frozen plasma may also be used. Obviously, avoidance of infection and use of appropriate antibiotics are also essential.

B. Transient hypogammaglobulinemia of infancy results when the onset of immunoglobulin synthesis, particularly IgG synthesis, is delayed beyond the norm. The cause is unknown but may be associated with a temporary deficiency of helper T (Th) cells.

     1. Clinical features. A normal infant is usually 5 to 6 months of age before new immunoglobulin is synthesized (IgG received through the placenta is catabolized faster than the new immunoglobulin is synthesized). However, infants with this disorder suffer recurrent pyogenic infections of, for example, the skin, meninges, or respiratory tract, usually caused by various gram-positive microorganisms until the situation is reversed, usually within 16 to 30 months of age.

     2. Treatment involves antibiotics, commercial gamma globulin, or both.

  C. Common variable hypogammaglobulinemia (acquired hypogammaglobulinemia) resembles Bruton's disease (see section III A) except that symptoms (e.g., repeated pyogenic infections) first appear when the patient is 20 to 30 years of age.

     1. Immunologic findings. The disorder is characterized by a high incidence of autoimmune disease.

       a. Although there is a normal number of circulating B cells, the ability to synthesize or secrete immunoglobulin, or both, is defective. The defect may be due to a population of Ts cells that suppress B-cell maturation and immunoglobulin production or secretion. The serum levels of immunoglobulins are low.

       b. T-cell function is usually intact, but it may be defective in some patients.

     2. Treatment is the same as that for Bruton's disease.

  D. Selective immunoglobulin deficiency (dysgammaglobulinemia) describes a decrease in the serum level of one or more immunoglobulins, but not all immunoglobulins, with normal or increased levels of the others. The most common form of this disorder is selective IgA deficiency.

     1. Clinical features include recurrent sinopulmonary infection, gastrointestinal disease, autoimmune disease, malignancy, and allergy. However, many individuals may be asymptomatic.

     2. Immunologic findings. There are slight serum levels of IgA, but serum levels of IgG and IgM are normal or increased. IgA-bearing B cells are present in normal numbers, but they are defective in their ability to synthesize or release IgA, possibly due to the presence of Ts cells in excessive numbers or due to hyperactivity of the Ts cells.

     3. Treatment consists of appropriate antibiotics. Administration of gamma globulin should be avoided since it might stimulate the formation of antibodies to IgA, which could trigger an anaphylactoid transfusion reaction.

IV. T-CELL DEFICIENCY DISORDERS

  A. DiGeorge syndrome (congenital thymic hypoplasia) is due to faulty development of the third and fourth pharyngeal pouches during embryogenesis, with resulting absence or hypoplasia of both the thymus and parathyroid glands.

     1. Clinical features

       a. DiGeorge syndrome is characterized by profoundly impaired T-cell function as manifested by recurrent infection with viral, fungal, protozoan, and certain bacterial agents. However, levels of immunoglobulins are normal.

       b. Hypoparathyroidism leads to hypocalcemia tetany. Thymus aplasia, or hypoplasia, results in cellular immunodeficiency. There is an abnormal facial appearance with a fish-shaped mouth and low-set ears. Cardiac anomalies are usually present.

     2. Immunologic findings. Lymphocytopenia is usual in these patients. T cells [i.e., E-rosetting cells and cells that respond to phytohemagglutinin (PHA)], are diminished in number. Delayed hypersensitivity reactions and ability to reject allografts are impaired. The levels of circulating antibody are low, at least to certain antigens, due to low numbers of Th cells.

     3. Treatment. Transplantation of a thymus from an aborted fetus can result in permanent reversal of the syndrome, with the production of functioning T cells. The fetus should not be older than 14 weeks gestation [to prevent graft-versus-host (GVH) disease], and the thymus can be either implanted or minced and injected. Hypocalcemia can be controlled by administration of calcium and vitamin D.

  B. Chronic mucocutaneous candidiasis is a syndrome of skin and mucous membrane infection with *Candida albicans*, which is associated with a rather unique defect in T-cell immunity.

     1. Immunologic findings. Although the total lymphocyte count appears to be normal and the presence of T cells is confirmed through their response to PHA and E-rosette tests, the ability of the cells to be activated by, or to produce macrophage migration-inhibition factor (MIF) in the presence of *Candida* antigen is impaired, although their response to other antigens may be normal. Likewise the delayed hypersensitivity skin reaction to *Candida* antigen is negative. The antibody response to *Candida* antigen is normal.

2. **Treatment**, with varying degrees of success, has been attempted with miconazole, amphotericin B, clotrimazole, transfer factor, and thymus transplantation.

V. COMBINED B-CELL AND T-CELL DEFICIENCY DISORDERS

A. **Severe combined immunodeficiency disease (SCID)** involves a combined defect in both humoral (B-cell) and cell-mediated (T-cell) immunity. Patients usually die within the first or second year of life from viral, bacterial, fungal, or protozoan infection. SCID may be inherited as an X-linked recessive or autosomal recessive disease.

1. **Immunologic findings**
   a. Classically SCID is associated with lymphopenia and hypoplasia of the thymus gland, as demonstrated on x-ray.
   b. There is an absence of T cells that form E-rosettes or respond to PHA or antigen. Patients are unable to respond to delayed hypersensitivity skin tests.
   c. Hypogammaglobulinemia and a lack of B cells and antibody response are characteristic.

2. **Treatment** with specific antibiotics and commercial gamma globulin is helpful, but successful immunologic reconstitution demands transplantation of histocompatible bone marrow. Transplantation of fetal liver and thymus has also shown promise. Isolation in a sterile environment ("bubble") has been used.

B. **Nezelof's syndrome** patients are susceptible to recurrent bacterial, fungal, viral, and protozoan infections.

1. **Immunologic findings.** The syndrome lacks uniformity in its clinical presentation, but rather consistent immunologic features include the following.
   a. There is a marked deficiency of T-cell immunity as manifested by reduction in cells that respond to PHA or antigen or that form E-rosettes. The ability to respond to delayed hypersensitivity skin tests is diminished.
   b. B-cell deficiency [i.e., low, normal, or elevated levels of specific immunoglobulin classes (dysgammaglobulinemia)] varies. The antibody response to specific antigens is usually low or absent.

2. **Treatment** with fetal thymus transplantation, thymic hormone administration, and transfer factor have been tried, with partial success. Administration of specific antibiotics and gamma globulin is useful.

C. **Wiskott-Aldrich syndrome** comprises a triad of features including thrombocytopenia, which is present at birth; eczema, which usually is present at the age of 1 year; and recurrent pyogenic infection (e.g., with *S. pneumoniae*, *Neisseria meningitidis*, or *H. influenzae*), starting after 6 months of age.

1. **Immunologic findings**
   a. There is a variable deficit in T-cell immunity. Levels of isohemagglutinins are low or absent.
   b. B cells are normal in number, although the B-cell deficit seems to be associated with a failure to make an antibody response to polysaccharide antigens. IgM levels are low, IgG levels are normal, and IgA and IgE levels are elevated.

2. **Treatment** involves vigorous use of antibiotics and bone marrow transplantation.

D. **Ataxia-telangiectasia** is an autosomal recessive disease and is characterized by uncoordinated muscle movements (ataxia) and dilatation of small blood vessels in the sclera of the eye (telangiectasia). It is associated with **repeated sinopulmonary infections** due to various viral and bacterial agents. The neurologic, endocrine, and vascular systems are involved.

1. **Immunologic findings.**
   a. There is selective IgA deficiency with variable abnormalities affecting other immunoglobulins and, occasionally, an inhibited antibody response to certain antigens.
   b. T-cell deficiency is variable.

2. **Treatment** of sinopulmonary infection with antibiotics is essential. Use of fetal thymus and bone marrow transplantation is of uncertain value.

E. Enzyme deficiencies have been reported to be the cause of at least some degree of combined immunodeficiency. Deficiencies of both **adenosine deaminase (ADA)** and **purine nucleoside phosphorylase (PNP)** are autosomal recessive traits. ADA and PNP are necessary for the purine salvage pathway.

$$\text{Adenosine} \xrightarrow{\text{ADA}} \text{Inosine} \xrightarrow{\text{PNP}} \text{Hypoxanthine}$$

  1. Features
  a. Adenosine is a substrate used by ADA. A deficiency of ADA causes adenosine accumulation, which inhibits lymphocyte function and interferes with energy metabolism.
  b. A deficiency of PNP is associated with T-cell immunodeficiency.

  2. Treatment with bone marrow transplantation has been used. In some patients, infusions of erythrocytes, which are high in ADA, have been helpful.

F. Acquired immune deficiency syndrome (AIDS) affects primarily, but not exclusively, male homosexuals, intravenous drug abusers, hemophiliacs, and other individuals who receive transfusions. It appears to be caused by a retrovirus, which formerly was referred to as human T-cell lymphotropic virus III (HTLV-III) or lymphadenopathy-associated virus (LAV) but now is designated human immunodeficiency virus (HIV).

  1. Clinical features. Patients demonstrate pronounced suppression of the immune system and development of Kaposi's sarcoma, severe opportunistic infection (e.g., with *Pneumocystis carinii, Mycobacterium avium-intracellulare,* or *Toxoplasma*), or both.

  2. Immunologic findings. Marked lymphopenia is associated with a reduction in the level of Th cells (identified by binding to T4 antibody) and resultant reversal of the Th:Ts (identified by binding with T8 antibody) ratio to less than 0.5 (normal $>$ 1.5). There is an impaired response of peripheral blood lymphocytes to PHA and specific antigens. Specific antibody production is impaired. The lymphocytes cannot produce the normal amount of interleukin-2, and the activity of natural killer (NK) cells is reduced.

  3. Treatment has, to date, been disappointing. Attempts to develop procedures for immunologic reversal are under investigation. Antimicrobial agents (e.g., trimethoprim–sulfamethoxazole) may be of value in the management of opportunistic infections.

VI. SECONDARY IMMUNODEFICIENCY.
Several conditions are associated with secondary immunodeficiency, which may be either transient or permanent and lead to increased susceptibility to opportunistic infection.

A. Measles is an example of a disease that induces immunosuppression. The infection induces a transient suppression of delayed hypersensitivity reactions. Lymphocytic response to antigens and mitogens is reduced. The number of circulating T cells is decreased. Similar effects may be seen following measles immunization.

B. Leprosy is another infection with associated immunodeficiency. Patients with lepromatous leprosy have an impaired ability to develop delayed hypersensitivity reactions. However, whether immunosuppression leads to or is caused by leprosy is not certain.

C. Tuberculosis and **coccidioidomycosis** are other examples. Both impair delayed hypersensitivity reactions.

VII. COMPLEMENT DEFICIENCY.
Deficiency of complement components and function has been associated with increased susceptibility to infection, autoimmune disease, and other disorders.

A. C$\overline{1}$ esterase inhibitor deficiency is linked with hereditary angioedema, a defect that is characterized by transient but recurrent localized edema. The skin, gastrointestinal tract, and respiratory tract may be affected. Laryngeal edema may be fatal. The defect leads to uncontrolled C$\overline{1}$s activity and resultant production of a kinin that increases capillary permeability.

B. C1q deficiency is reported to be associated with hypogammaglobulinemia, SCID, and repeated infections. The level of C1q has been reported to be about 50% of normal levels in affected individuals.

C. C2 and C4 deficiencies can cause a disorder similar to systemic lupus erythematosus (SLE), possibly due to failure of complement-dependent mechanisms to eliminate immune complexes.

D. C3 deficiencies can result in severe life-threatening infections, particularly with *N. meningitidis* and *S. pneumoniae*. Absence of the C3 component means that chemotactic fragments will not be generated, with resultant impaired opsonization.

E. C5 deficiency leads to increased susceptibility to bacterial infection associated with impaired chemotaxis.

F. C6, C7, and C8 deficiencies are associated with increased susceptibility to meningococcal and gonococcal infections, since complement-mediated lysis of *Neisseria* is a major control mechanism of immunity.

STUDY QUESTIONS

Directions: Each question below contains five suggested answers. Choose the **one best** response to each question.

RIST   Test. for → Total IGE

1. Bruton's hypogammaglobulinemia is indicative of a deficiency of what cell type?

(A) B cell
(B) Macrophage
(C) T cell
(D) Monocyte
(E) Neutrophil

2. Job's syndrome is thought to be due to

↑ IGE

(A) a B-cell deficit
(B) suppressed IgE production
(C) a defect in macrophage killing
(D) a defect in neutrophil chemotaxis
(E) suppressed IgA production

a defect in neutrophil function → chronic granulomatous

Directions: Each question below contains four suggested answers of which **one or more** is correct. Choose the answer

A	if **1, 2, and 3** are correct
B	if **1 and 3** are correct
C	if **2 and 4** are correct
D	if **4** is correct
E	if **1, 2, 3, and 4** are correct

3. Chronic granulomatous disease is due to which of the following immunodeficiency conditions?

(1) Hypocomplementemia
(2) A defect in T-cell function
(3) A defect in B-cell function
(4) A defect in neutrophil function

4. Transplantation of the thymus gland from an aborted fetus to an immunodeficient neonate has been beneficial in which of the following immunodeficiency disorders?

(1) Chédiak-Higashi syndrome
(2) DiGeorge Syndrome
(3) Bruton's hypogammaglobulinemia
(4) Severe combined immunodeficiency disease (SCID)

Directions: The group of questions below consists of lettered choices followed by several numbered items. For each numbered item select the **one** lettered choice with which it is **most** closely associated. Each lettered choice may be used once, more than once, or not at all.

Questions 5–9

For each immunodeficiency disorder listed to the right, select the characteristic that is most closely associated with it.

(A) Selective IgA deficiency plus variable T-cell deficiency
(B) Marked lymphopenia associated with reversal of helper:suppressor cell (Th:Ts) ratio
(C) Clinical features similar to those of systemic lupus erythematosus (SLE)
(D) Defective development of all bone marrow stem cells
(E) Normal numbers of circulating B cells but defective synthesis or secretion of immunoglobulin, or both

5. Acquired immune deficiency syndrome (AIDS)
6. Common variable hypogammaglobulinemia
7. C2 deficiency → *lupus → 85% in ♀ due to Estrogen*
8. Ataxia-telangiectasia
9. Reticular dysgenesis

ANSWERS AND EXPLANATIONS

1. The answer is A. (*III A 1 b*) Patients with Bruton's hypogammaglobulinemia are deficient in B cells and plasma cells and hence have low serum levels of all classes of immunoglobulins. T-cell and phagocytic function are normal.

2. The answer is D. (*II B 4*) Job's syndrome (hyper-IgE syndrome) is characterized by "cold" staphylococcal abscesses, chronic eczema, and extremely high serum levels of IgE. It is related to defective neutrophil chemotaxis. Neutrophil ingestion and killing appear to be normal.

3. The answer is D (4). (*II B 1*) Chronic granulomatous disease reflects an inability of neutrophils to respond to phagocytosis with the normal oxidative burst and apparently it is due to reduction in intracellular reduced nicotinamide adenine dinucleotide (NADH) or nicotinamide adenine dinucleotide phosphate (NADPH). There is also decreased iodination and superoxide anion production and absence of cytochrome b. The result is suppression of intracellular killing of ingested microorganisms. B-cell, T-cell, and NK-cell functions, as well as complement levels, are generally normal. The mortality rate can be reduced considerably by early diagnosis and aggressive therapy.

4. The answer is C (2, 4). (*IV A 3; V A 2*) Patients with DiGeorge syndrome (congenital thymic hypoplasia) are markedly deficient in thymic tissue due to faulty development of the third and fourth pharyngeal pouches during embryogenesis. This results in profoundly impaired T-cell function. Treatment via fetal thymus transplantation can result in permanent reversal and the production of functioning T cells. Severe combined immunodeficiency disease results from a combined defect in both B-cell and T-cell immunity. Treatment consists of transplantation of histocompatible bone marrow. In the absence of a suitable bone marrow donor, fetal thymus or liver has been transplanted with some success.

5–9. The answers are: 5-B, 6-E, 7-C, 8-A, 9-D. (*II A 1 c; III C 1 a; V D, F; VII C*) Acquired immune deficiency syndrome (AIDS) appears to be caused by a retrovirus, human immunodeficiency virus (HIV), that causes a marked reduction in helper T (Th) cells and a marked reversal of the helper:suppressor cell (Th:Ts) ratio to less than 0.5 (normal > 1.5). This leads to pronounced suppression of the immune system with resultant susceptibility to opportunistic infections.

Common variable hypogammaglobulinemia is characterized by normal levels of circulating B cells, but the ability to synthesize or secrete immunoglobulin, or both, is defective. The defect may be due to a population of Ts cells that suppress B-cell maturation.

A deficiency in complement component C2 may manifest itself as a disorder similar to systemic lupus erythematosus (SLE), possibly due to failure of complement-dependent mechanisms to eliminate immune complexes.

Ataxia-telangiectasia, an inherited immune deficiency, is characterized by uncoordinated muscle movements (ataxia) and dilatated small blood vessels in the sclera of the eye (telangiectasia). Immune deficits include variable T-cell deficiency, selective IgA deficiency with variable abnormalities in other immunoglobulins, and an occasional inhibited antibody response to certain antigens.

Reticular dysgenesis, an inherited defect, also referred to as severe combined immunodeficiency disease (SCID) with leukopenia, results from defective development of all bone marrow stem cells, including myeloid precursors.

12
Immunogenetics and Transplantation Immunology

I. INTRODUCTION

A. The transfer of normal tissue between genetically identical individuals (i.e., between identical twins; between animals of the same inbred line) is the grafting of **syngeneic tissue** (**syngrafts; isografts**). Generally, isografts and **autografts** (i.e., grafts removed from and placed on the same organism) survive for an indefinite period of time.

B. Transplantation of normal tissue between genetically different individuals of the same species is referred to as **allogeneic** (**allografts; homografts**). **Xenogeneic grafts** are those transferred between animals of two different species. Allogeneic and xenogeneic transplantation results in an immune rejection phenomenon, of a lesser or greater degree, which may or may not be prevented or aborted by the use of immunosuppressive agents.

C. The **histocompatibility antigens**—a term that is synonymous with transplantation antigens—determine compatibility or incompatibility of transplanted tissue. It is these antigens that induce the immune response in the host that is necessary for the rejection of the tissue.

D. Incompatibility of the red blood cell system cannot be violated with the expectation of graft survival. The **ABO antigens** of the red blood cell system act as strong transplantation antigens.

II. HISTOCOMPATIBILITY GENE COMPLEX

A. Immunogenetics is the study of genetic variations in individuals, and includes the study of the genetic factors that control the immune response as well as the genetics of the antigenic composition of the individual. Immunogenicity is the capacity of an antigen to provoke an immune response.

   1. The major histocompatibility genes determine the specificity of tissue antigenicity and, therefore, transplantation compatibility between donor and recipient.

      a. The major histocompatibility genes of mice are found on chromosome 17; this gene complex is termed **H-2**.

      b. In humans, the major histocompatibility genes reside in a region of chromosome 6. These genes code for the histocompatibility antigens termed **human leukocyte antigens (HLA)**. The HLA gene complex is presented schematically in Figure 12-1.

   2. Histocompatibility antigens are products of genes of the **major histocompatibility complex (MHC)**. These antigens are found in high concentrations on lymphocytes; they also occur on other nucleated cells of the body (e.g., macrophages and hepatocytes), including leukocytes.

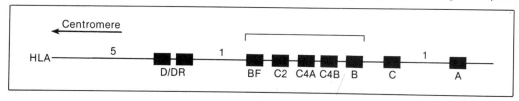

Figure 12-1. Schematic representation of the major histocompatibility gene complex in humans. *Numbers* indicate the approximate map distance between loci. Loci associated with certain complement components (i.e., C2, C4, and factor B of the alternative pathway) are bracketed; the order of these loci is not known. The immune response (Ir) genes are close to the D locus. (Adapted from Klein J: *Immunology the Science of Self-Nonself Discrimination*. New York, John Wiley, 1982, p 284.)

3. Each gene of the HLA complex is highly **polymorphic**. The genes that dictate the nature of these antigens occur in allelic form (i.e., multiple genes may occur at a single locus). Since many alleles exist at each locus, the genes encode many histocompatibility antigens. These genes are **codominant** in expression. This means that in a heterozygous individual (i.e., having different alleles at corresponding loci of the two chromosomes) both alleles are expressed (Fig. 12-2). Therefore, the antigens encoded by these genes are present on the tissue cells.

    a. If two chromosomes are present, and each chromosome has an A and a B locus, a maximum of four gene products (antigens) and, therefore, four HLA antigens, can be specified.

    b. If the alleles of the loci on both chromosomes are identical, only one HLA antigen is specified by the corresponding loci.

    c. Therefore, depending on the genes present, a person may have two, three, or four different HLA antigens determined by the A and B loci.

B. Classification of HLA molecules. Essentially, there are two classes of molecules encoded by genes of the MHC. Both classes of antigens are surface components of the cell and are composed of alpha and beta chains. They are 90% protein and 10% carbohydrate. (The molecular configuration of a histocompatibility antigen is presented in Figure 12-3.)

    1. General considerations

      a. HLA antigens are controlled by a complex of genes at loci closely linked on chromosome 6. The antigens coded for by these loci include HLA-A, HLA-B, HLA-C, and HLA-D/DR. Each locus has several alleles: A, B, and D/DR have approximately 20 allelic forms each; locus C has 8. Provisional alleles are designated with a "**w**," which is dropped when the antigen is proved to be truly new.

      b. Genes found in the HLA locus include **immune response (Ir) genes**. Specific Ir genes are found in inbred lines of animals, indicating that the response to a particular antigen is genetically controlled.

    2. Class I antigens. The function of class I (and class II) antigens is not really clear. Both class I and class II molecules are important in controlling immunologic defense. Class I antigens are involved in the **effector phase of cell-mediated cytolysis (CMC)**: There must be identity with the T-cell target cell. Expression of cell-mediated immunity and killing of, for example, virus-modified target cells can only occur if the target cell and the T cell have the **same** class I MHC antigen in their membranes.

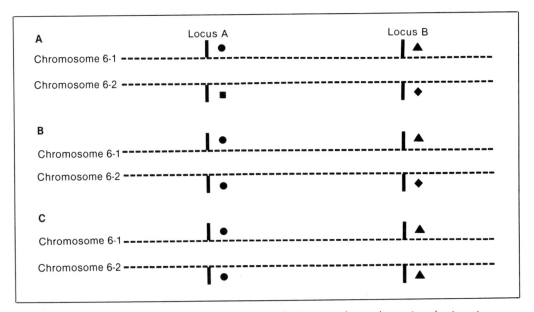

Figure 12-2. Schematic representation of chromosome 6. In the HLA complex, each gene is codominant in expression (i.e., in an individual having different alleles at corresponding loci of the two chromosomes, both alleles are expressed). ●, ■, ▲, ◆ = HLA antigens expressed by each locus on both chromosomes. In situation *A*, four different antigens are expressed (●■▲◆); in situation *B*, three different antigens are expressed (●▲◆); in situation *C*, two different antigens are expressed (●▲).

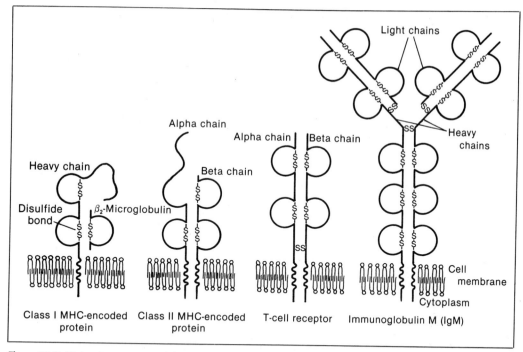

Figure 12-3. Molecular structures of the class I major histocompatibility complex (MHC) encoded protein, the class II protein, the T-cell receptor, and the immunoglobulin molecule. Note the structural similarity; the molecules also share similar sequences of amino acids. The molecules are characterized by loops made up of about 70 amino acids within each chain. (Adapted from Marrack P, Kappler J: The T cell and its receptor. *Sci Am* 254:36–45, 1986.)

a. The three MHC-encoded class I antigens are HLA-A, HLA-B, and HLA-C, which are found on all nucleated human cells. Each gene is highly polymorphic, with many alleles existing for each locus. Structurally, the class I antigens are two polypeptide chains held together noncovalently.
  (1) The heavy chain (44,000 daltons) has antigenic specificity and is anchored in the cell membrane.
  (2) The other chain is a nonpolymorphic β_2-microglobulin of 12,000 daltons.
b. HLA-A and HLA-B antigens are the principal antigens recognized by the host during the process of graft rejection, thus their designation as major transplantation antigens. Graft rejection is principally in the province of T cells (with some B-cell participation). In CMC, the in vitro correlate of graft rejection, HLA-A and HLA-B antigens are the target antigens recognized by the cytotoxic T cells.
c. Class I antigens are also involved in **MHC restriction** of CMC of virus-infected cells.
  (1) A viral antigen may combine with a class I antigen on the cell surface. Thus, the T cell recognizes it within the context of a class I antigen.
  (2) The response mounted by the host is restricted to the elimination of cells bearing the virus–class I antigen complex. The T cells do not kill cells bearing the same viral antigen and a different class I antigen, nor do they kill cells bearing a different viral antigen and the same class I antigen.

3. Class II antigens [immune response-associated (Ia) antigens]
  a. The class II antigens are HLA-D/DR antigens (D, DP, DQ, and DR), which are found chiefly on the surfaces of immunocompetent cells, including macrophages, monocytes, resting T cells (in low amounts), activated T cells, and, particularly, B cells. The class II antigens consist of two chains, alpha (34,000 daltons) and beta (29,000 daltons), which are joined on the cell surface by noncovalent bonds. The beta chain is polymorphic. Each chain consists of two extracellular domains (α_1, α_2, β_1, β_2), a connecting peptide, a transmembrane region, and a cytoplasmic tail. The chains are encoded in four closely linked gene clusters (D, DP, DQ, and DR) found on chromosome 6.
  b. The **mixed lymphocyte reaction (MLR)** is often used to define and detect class II antigens. The reaction is a response of T cells to antigens on B cells. Lymphocytes are stimulated to divide when those from one individual are cultured with those from another individual.

Small lymphocytes are transformed into blast cells. Histocompatibility varies inversely with the number of blast cells (see section II C 3).
c. Class II antigens are thought to be the antigens principally responsible for the **graft-versus-host (GVH) reaction**, which is an in vivo correlate of the MLR.
d. Sensitization occurs when an immune response is stimulated upon first exposure to an antigen. The immune system is prepared for a stronger response when it is again exposed to that same antigen. The HLA-D/DR antigens have been implicated as activators in the sensitization phase of CMC. (This is another case of MHC restriction. In this instance, there must be identity of class II antigens before effective interaction and immune response induction can occur.) This is in contrast to the **effector phase** of CMC (in which effector cells carry out the killing of target cells), where HLA class I molecules are targets.
e. The HLA-D/DR antigens have a role in antigen presentation by macrophages to T cells and in T-cell interaction with B cells.
f. Many diseases have been associated with molecules of the MHC, and most HLA-associated diseases are connected to the HLA-D/DR haplotypes, particularly the DR and DQ loci. For example, several autoimmune diseases, such as systemic lupus erythematosus, occur more frequently in individuals with the HLA-DR3 antigen. HLA antigen occurrence and its association with some autoimmune diseases are presented in Table 12-1.

4. Class III antigens. There are loci on chromosome 6 that are associated with certain complement components (i.e., C2, C4, and factor B of the alternative pathway). Class III antigens are not involved in either immune responsiveness or graft rejection.

C. Histocompatibility testing

1. Sources of cells and typing sera
a. The best cells for detecting HLA antigens are peripheral blood lymphocytes and lymphocytes obtained from lymph nodes, spleen, or thymus, which are used because of their availability and because they have the highest concentration of HLA antigens on the cell surface.
b. The majority of the HLA antigens are coded for at the A, B, and C loci. All of these class I molecules can be identified by serologic procedures. The sources of the typing sera used in the cytotoxicity assay are as follows.
(1) Multiparous women. During pregnancy, fetal lymphoid cells can cross the placenta into the mother's circulation and sensitize her (much like Rh sensitization, although no fetal disease has been associated with HLA sensitization; see Chapter 9, section III C 1 b). The fetal antigens that are derived from the father's genetic contribution will be foreign to the mother.
(2) Patients who have received multiple transfusions. The white blood cells and platelets in the transfused blood provide the sensitizing antigens.
(3) Volunteers who have been sensitized by blood transfusions, white blood cell inoculations, or tissue grafts
(4) Patients who have rejected a transplanted kidney

2. In the **lymphocytotoxicity test**, purified lymphocytes plus various test sera are allowed to react. If a test serum contains an antibody to one of the HLA antigens on the cell, it will fix to it. Complement is then added, and incubation is continued. The cell membranes disintegrate, causing cell death. Dead cells are stained with trypan blue or eosin, which is specifically taken up into damaged or dying cells. Because live cells do not take up the dye, it can be demonstrated whether a particular test serum–complement combination is cytotoxic for the lymphocytes.

3. The **blastogenesis assay** (the MLR; see section II B 3 b) uses DNA synthesis to detect the histo-

Table 12-1. Association between HLA-D/DR Alleles and Autoimmune Diseases

Disease	Antigen	Relative Risk*
Multiple sclerosis	HLA-DR2	4
Systemic lupus erythematosus	HLA-DR3	6
Myasthenia gravis	HLA-DR3	3
Rheumatoid arthritis	HLA-DR4	4
Hashimoto's thyroiditis	HLA-DR5	3

*Disease risk of individuals who bear the antigen as opposed to those who do not (e.g., if an individual is DR2 positive, he is four times more likely to develop multiple sclerosis than if he is DR2 negative).

compatibility antigens dictated by the HLA-D/DR locus. Over 20 antigens are encoded on this locus, and all can be detected by the MLR. Some (the DR) can also be identified by serologic assays. The blastogenesis assay is usually done in a one-way procedure (i.e., only one of the cells in the mixture can respond). Lymphocyte division is prevented by irradiating the donor's cells or treating them with mitomycin C, which cross-links DNA. Thus, the cells cannot undergo blast transformation but can still act as stimulating cells. The recipient's cells may or may not respond. If there are several potential donor–recipient pairs or several donors, the donor chosen should have lymphocytes that stimulate the recipient the **least**.

D. Inheritance and expression of blood group antigens

1. Blood group antigens are genetically determined antigens found on the surface of red blood cells. They are biologically significant because they are present on other tissues in addition to blood (e.g., the kidney) and thus are associated with the determination of histocompatibility.

2. **Blood type** is the antigenic **phenotype**, which is the **serologic expression of the blood group genes**. In this instance, the term "phenotype" refers to the red blood cell characteristics that differentiate one individual or group from another individual or group.
   a. Various phenotypes are determined by different gene combinations. The four antigenic types (blood groups) of the ABO system are A, B, AB, and O.
   b. The A, B, and O genes occur as pairs on the two sets of chromosomes in the nucleus of all human cells except the sperm and ovum (Table 12-2).
      (1) People in either the A or B blood group can be either homozygous (AA, BB) or heterozygous (AO, BO).
      (2) Those in the O blood group are homozygous (OO).
      (3) People in the AB blood group are heterozygous (AB).

3. The ABO blood group is a system of antigens with allelic genes. The ABO antigens are under the influence of four loci, ABO, H, Se, and Le.
   a. The ABO gene has three alleles, A, B, and O; A and B are dominant over O.
      (1) The A and B genes control the formation of transferase enzymes which add specific monosaccharide units to an existing oligosaccharide core; A transferase adds *N*-acetylgalactosamine, and B transferase adds galactose. This is not true of the O gene, which is not a true gene as it codes for no product.
      (2) O cells do have a distinctive antigen, which is referred to as an **H antigen** because it is a heterophil antigen.
   b. The H antigen is the oligosaccharide core and functions as the precursor to the A and B antigens. Products of the A and B genes convert the H substance to A and B antigens.
   c. The H gene codes for an enzyme that is involved in the synthesis of the oligosaccharide core.
   d. The Se gene is present in individuals who secrete the ABO blood group antigens. In the majority of the population, the ABO antigens are found in a soluble form in body secretions such as saliva, urine, and serum. About 25% of the population are **nonsecretors**.
   e. The **Lewis antigen** is specified by the Le gene, which, like the H gene, segregates independently from A, B, and O. The Le antigen appears to arise from the same precursor as the ABO antigens, and it appears to be a precursor of the H antigen.

III. WORKUP OF THE DONOR–RECIPIENT COMBINATION

A. First, ABO blood group compatibility must be met.

B. Histocompatibility (HLA) antigen typing must be performed.

C. The recipient's serum must be tested for the presence of preformed antibodies against the donor's tissues.

1. These antibodies can be formed following multiple blood transfusions, following an earlier transplantation, or in a woman who has had several pregnancies [see section II C 1 b (1)].

Table 12-2. ABO Blood Group Genetics and Occurrence

Phenotype	Genotype	Occurrence (%)*
A	AA or AO	40
B	BB or BO	10
O	OO	45
AB	AB	5

*Figures represent percentage of United States' population.

2. A **lymphocytotoxicity test** is performed (see section II C 2). A number of samples of the patient's serum are collected over a period of time. All of the serum samples must be cross-matched against the donor's lymphocytes because the titer of the antibodies may change and, thus, be detectable only in one serum sample. If even one cross-matching kills the donor's lymphocytes, transplantation is not performed.

D. When the donor–recipient pair is comprised of HLA-identical siblings, the MLR is used to determine if the donor cells stimulate the reaction (see section II B 3 b).

1. When HLA-identical siblings are used for kidney transplantation, more than 90% of the transplants have a 5-year survival rate.

2. When two antigens match, the graft survival rate is 70% to 85%.

3. When more than two antigens are mismatched, the chances for graft survival are considerably lower.

4. In cadaver grafts, regardless of matching, the 5-year survival rate is 33% to 50% for kidney transplants.

IV. HOST RESPONSE TO TRANSPLANTATION

A. At least **three types of rejection reactions** can take place following transplantation.

1. Hyperacute rejection. In this situation, the recipient has preformed antibodies, and as soon as the vascular supplies between the recipient and the donor organ are linked, the antibodies start attacking the organ. In certain cases, the organ will fail to show any blood flow. There is a rapid vascular spasm and vascular occlusion, and the organ will never be perfused by the recipient's blood. This rejection pattern can occur when the donor and recipient have not been matched for ABO blood group antigens.

2. Acute or accelerated rejection. Acute rejection is believed to be due to sensitized lymphocytes. This type of reaction occurs 10 to 30 days after transplantation. Since the recipient has not been previously sensitized, it takes time for him to develop sensitized lymphocytes, which then increase in number and attack the graft. This is the typical picture of a cell-mediated immune response. The graft (especially around small blood vessels) is infiltrated with small lymphocytes and mononuclear cells along with some granulocytes, causing destruction of the transplanted tissue.

3. Chronic rejection. There is a slow loss of tissue function over a period of months or years in chronic rejection. This may be a cellular immune response, an antibody response, or a combination of the two. The antigens that evoke chronic rejection may be weak antigens of the HLA system or antigens in minor histocompatibility loci such as those on the Y chromosome.

B. Immunologic tolerance and enhancement can be achieved in the graft recipient.

1. Suppressor T (Ts) cells may be induced that down-regulate the graft rejection arm of the immune response. These are specific to the particular histocompatibility antigens of the graft.
  a. Tolerance to foreign histocompatibility antigens can be induced in fetal animals through injection of tissue containing foreign antigens.
  b. Tolerance may be induced in human transplantation recipients by giving large-volume blood transfusions of the donor's blood prior to the transplantation procedure.

2. In contrast to immunologic tolerance, immunologic enhancement is the enhancement of graft survival by specific antibodies. These graft-specific antibodies interfere with the destructive action of cytotoxic T (Tc) cells. The antibodies are most likely growth-promoting (as opposed to cytotoxic) immunoglobulins, particularly IgA or IgG4 noncomplement-fixing antibodies.

3. Immunologic tolerance or, at least, graft-specific immunosuppression may occur, either as a result of Ts-cell development, helper T (Th)-cell depletion, or terminal (exhaustive) differentiation of B cells or Tc-cell precursors.

V. POSTOPERATIVE MANAGEMENT. All transplant recipients require immunosuppressive therapy primarily directed at blocking the induction or expression of cell-mediated immunity. The only exception is a case in which the donor and recipient are identical twins.

A. Immunosuppressive drugs

1. Corticosteroids are used for maintenance therapy or are given in a bolus at the time of a rejection crisis.

2. Antimetabolites and alkylating agents are also used.
   a. Azathioprine is a commonly used antimetabolite.
   b. Cyclophosphamide (a cyclized nitrogen mustard) is a popular alkylating agent.

3. Cyclosporine (formerly called cyclosporin A), an antibiotic produced by the fungus *Trichoderma inflatum*, is very effective in inhibiting the T-cell arm of the rejection process. It does not seem to affect B-cell activities.

4. Antilymphocyte globulin or antithymocyte globulin is used almost universally today in some centers as a postoperative (for approximately 2 weeks) prophylactic agent, and it is used in many centers in the management of acute rejection episodes. It promotes graft survival.

B. With the use of high doses of immunosuppressive drugs, infection often occurs. About 25% of the deaths that occur in kidney transplantations are due to sepsis.

C. Patients with transplants also have a high rate of **spontaneous malignancy**.

   1. About 6% of all transplant patients develop a malignancy. Some are common malignancies such as carcinoma of the skin; however, about one half of the malignancies are lymphomas and reticuloendothelial cell sarcomas.

   2. This excessive susceptibility to malignancy may be explained by a drug-induced impairment in immunosurveillance. Ordinarily, the immune system is policing the body for mutated cancerous cells. When the immune system is suppressed, these cells are allowed to escape and proliferate.

VI. SPECIAL GRAFT SITUATIONS

A. Privileged tissues

   1. Immunologically privileged tissues are tissues from different anatomical locations that are not rejected no matter where they are transplanted. Included among these tissues are bone, cartilage, tendon, and sections of major blood vessels. The fetus can also be considered privileged tissue.

   2. The use of nonvascularized tissue as the graft ordinarily eliminates immune rejection. For example, the **cornea** can restore vision when transplanted under acceptable surgical conditions and when the vascular bed is not damaged. However, if the cornea is placed in vascularized tissue or if there is trauma at the site of transplantation with inflammation and vascularization, the grafted cornea is rejected.

B. Privileged sites. Certain areas such as the brain, the anterior chamber of the eye, and the cheek pouch of hamsters are regarded as **privileged sites**. These sites tolerate grafting without sensitization of the recipient. This is most likely due to the dearth or complete lack of lymphatic drainage in surrounding tissues.

C. Graft-versus-host (GVH) disease

   1. When an immunologically competent graft is transplanted into an immunologically compromised host, the graft tissue can mount an immunologic attack on the recipient. This is termed **graft rejection of the host**.

   2. GVH disease involves mainly the skin, alimentary tract, and liver. It is not a consideration with heart or kidney transplantation, although it is a major factor in limiting allogeneic bone marrow transplantation in humans.
   a. The problem occurs when there is an antigen difference between the donor and the immunologically compromised recipient. If the transplanted bone marrow lacks specific histocompatibility antigens that the host has, the bone marrow can produce immunologically competent lymphocytes that become sensitized to the recipient's antigens. Bone marrow transplantation should only be done between people who are histocompatible—preferably between histoidentical siblings.
   b. If the T cells are removed from the bone marrow by in vitro manipulation, such as use of antitheta serum plus complement, the incidence and severity of GVH reactions can be markedly reduced.

   3. The GVH reaction in humans is characterized by liver abnormalities and by a skin rash that resembles measles, as well as by diarrhea, wasting, and death.

STUDY QUESTIONS

Directions: Each question below contains five suggested answers. Choose the **one best** response to each question.

1. Several types of immunologic rejection reactions can occur following organ transplantation. The rejection reaction that is caused by the presence of preformed antibodies in the recipient is referred to as

(A) acute
(B) hyperacute
(C) chronic
(D) immediate
(E) accelerated

2. Class I HLA antigens can be described as

(A) cell surface proteins that contain HLA-A, HLA-B, and HLA-C determinants
(B) involved in macrophage interactions with B cells
(C) complement components
(D) involved in the activator phase of cell-mediated cytolysis (CMC)
(E) principally responsible for the graft-versus-host (GVH) reaction

3. As compared to T cells, B cell membranes are rich in

(A) class I antigens
(B) class II antigens
(C) class III antigens
(D) HLA-B antigens
(E) complement activating antigens

4. Under which of the following conditions do graft-versus-host (GVH) reactions occur?

(A) When the graft is contaminated with gram-negative microorganisms
(B) When tumor tissues are grafted
(C) When viable T cells are present in the graft
(D) When the graft has histocompatibility antigens not found in the recipient
(E) When the graft is pretreated with antilymphocyte serum

5. Antilymphocyte globulin and antithymocyte globulin are effective in suppressing allograft rejection because of their ability to

(A) suppress cell-mediated immunity
(B) suppress humoral immunity
(C) block lymphocyte transformation
(D) react with antigens in the graft
(E) mimic anti-idiotype antibodies induced during graft rejection

6. Efficient T-cell–mediated killing of virus-infected cells requires major histocompatibility complex (MHC) antigen compatibility (identity) with

(A) ABO blood group antigens
(B) Rh blood group antigens
(C) class I antigens
(D) class II antigens
(E) class III antigens

7. All of the following are considered to be privileged tissues for grafting EXCEPT

(A) the cornea
(B) bone
(C) bone marrow
(D) cartilage
(E) fetus

Directions: Each question below contains four suggested answers of which **one or more** is correct. Choose the answer

A if **1, 2, and 3** are correct
B if **1 and 3** are correct
C if **2 and 4** are correct
D if **4** is correct
E if **1, 2, 3, and 4** are correct

8. HLA-A and HLA-B antigens can be described as

(1) class I antigens found on most nucleated cells of the body
(2) the targets recognized by the host during graft rejection
(3) being involved in major histocompatibility complex (MHC) restriction of cell-mediated cytolysis (CMC)
(4) composed of an alpha chain, noncovalently associated with β_2-microglobulin

E

9. Donor–recipient compatibility is determined through the evaluation of which of the antigenic systems listed?

(1) Class I HLA antigens
(2) ABO blood group
(3) Class II HLA antigens
(4) Antibodies to donor lymphocytes

E

10. Antigens that act as transplantation barriers include   *don't accept graft*

(1) ABO antigens
(2) class I antigens
(3) class II antigens
(4) class III antigens

A

Directions: For each numbered item below, select the one lettered choice with which it is most closely associated. Each lettered choice may be used once, more than once, or not at all. Choose the answer

A if the item is associated with **(A) only**
B if the item is associated with **(B) only**
C if the item is associated with **both (A) and (B)**
D if the item is associated with **neither (A) nor (B)**

11. Immune response (Ir) genes can be characterized by

(A) their association with the major histocompatibility (MHC) locus
(B) exertion of their control through B cells
(C) both
(D) neither

12. An antibody response to foreign tissue is suppressed by T cells in which of the following phenomena?

(A) Immune tolerance
(B) Immune enhancement
(C) Both
(D) Neither

13. Immunologically based chronic graft rejection may be caused by

(A) specifically sensitized lymphocytes
(B) humoral antibodies
(C) both
(D) neither

14. The β_2-microglobulin component of class I antigens resembles an

(A) L chain
(B) H chain
(C) both
(D) neither

ANSWERS AND EXPLANATIONS

1. The answer is B. *(IV A 1)* Hyperacute rejection of a transplanted organ occurs when preformed antibodies attack the donor organ, causing a rapid vascular spasm and vascular occlusion and lack of organ perfusion by the recipient's blood. This may occur with ABO blood group mismatch, when a donor organ containing blood group A or group B antigens is transplanted into a patient who has preformed anti-A antibodies or anti-B antibodies. A similar hyperacute rejection reaction can result with HLA antigen mismatch, when the recipient has preformed antibodies to an HLA antigen in the donor's serum.

2. The answer is A. *(II B 2, 3 c, d)* The cell surface membrane proteins that contain HLA-A, HLA-B, and HLA-C determinants are called class I antigens. These antigens are involved in effector cell recognition of target tissues. Class II antigens are also coded for in the major histocompatibility complex (MHC) and are involved in antigen-processing macrophage interactions with B cells and with T-cell–B-cell interactions. There is a phenomenon referred to as MHC restriction, which means that the macrophage must bear an identical class II antigen to that expressed on the B-cell membrane. Class III HLA antigens are not involved in histocompatibility but are complement components, specifically C2, C4, and factor B.

3. The answer is B. *(II B 2 a, 3 a)* B-cell membranes are rich in class II HLA antigens, which also are found in macrophage membranes as well as in the membranes of activated peripheral blood lymphocytes. Class I HLA antigens are found on all lymphocytes and macrophages—on most nucleated cells.

4. The answer is C. *(VI C; see also Chapter 8)* Graft-versus-host (GVH) reactions are an expression of T-cell function, and removal of T cells by treatment with T3 or T11 antiserum before bone marrow engraftment should prevent a reaction from taking place. The presence of contaminating microbes in a graft would certainly contribute to rejection of the graft but not to graft rejection of the recipient. Tumors are dedifferentiated tissues that cannot participate in GVH reactions. The recipient must have HLA antigens that are not found in the donor in order for the GVH reaction to occur.

5. The answer is A. *(V A 4)* Antilymphocyte and antithymocyte globulins suppress cell-mediated immunity, thus promoting graft survival. Antilymphocyte serum might also suppress antibody formation. Lymphocyte transformation could actually be triggered by antilymphocyte serum (in the absence of complement) if the serum was directed to the proper membrane component [e.g., to the phytohemagglutinin (PHA) or lipopolysaccharide (LPS) receptors]. Noncomplement-fixing antibodies could react with transplantation antigens and block cytotoxic T-cell interaction with the grafted tissue.

6. The answer is C. *(II B 2)* Class I antigens (i.e., HLA-A, -B, and -C) are involved in cell-mediated immune functions. The target cell and the cytotoxic lymphocyte must be identical with regard to the HLA antigens coded at the A and B loci. Class II homology is a prerequisite for the cellular interactions that occur during the inductive phase of an immune response.

7. The answer is C. *(VI A, C)* The cornea, bone, and cartilage are privileged tissue and do not evoke an immune response in a graft recipient. The fetus does not induce a response in the mother at any time during pregnancy, although it has been theorized that the induction of labor may be due to an immunologically based rejection episode. Bone marrow transplantation is particularly difficult and dangerous, due to the high probability of rejection, particularly graft versus host (GVH) disease.

8. The answer is E (all). *(II B 2 a–c)* HLA antigens coded for by the A, B, and C loci are class I antigens, the specificity of which is determined by polymorphism in the alpha (heavy) chain which is associated with a nonpolymorphic β_2-microglobulin on the cell membrane. They are also involved in major histocompatibility complex (MHC) restriction, and cytotoxic T cell–target cell interactions can only occur if there is homology in the class I antigen makeup of the two cells.

9. The answer is E (all). *(II C 2; III A, B, C, D)* The ABO blood group is a system of antigens that is significant in the determination of histocompatibility. ABO blood group compatibility must exist between donor and recipient; crossing the blood group barrier compromises graft survival.

HLA antigen typing must be performed in the evaluation of donor–recipient compatibility. This is done through cytotoxicity assays, including the lymphocytotoxicity test, in which purified lymphocytes and various test sera are allowed to react and dye is introduced into the test medium. When cytotoxic antibodies react with cell surface antigens, the cell membrane disintegrates and the cell dies. Viable cells do not permit dyes such as trypan blue or eosin to enter the cytoplasm; the dye is specifically taken up by damaged and dying cells. Serum suitable for histocompatibility typing is obtained from multiparous women, the recipients of many blood transfusions, and patients who have rejected a transplanted kidney. A similar action could occur if serum from a sensitized recipient were allowed to react with donor lymphocytes. Such a reaction would negate the use of that particular donor.

In the mixed lymphocyte reaction (MLR), lymphocytes from both the prospective donor and the recipient are cultured and observed for reactions. Histocompatibility is assumed to exist if blastogenesis does not occur.

10. The answer is A (1, 2, 3). *(II B 1, 2, 3, D 1; III A, B)* Transplantation antigens that function as barriers to the acceptance of a graft include class I and class II HLA antigens of the major histocompatibility complex (MHC) plus the blood group ABO system. Class III HLA antigens are serum proteins; specifically, the complement factors, C2, C4, and factor B of the alternative pathway.

11. The answer is C. *(II B 1 b, 3 e)* Immune response (Ir) genes code for the production of class II major histocompatibility complex (MHC) antigens referred to as immune response-associated (Ia) antigens. Ir genes are important in the interaction of the antigen-presenting macrophage with the antigen-specific B cell. The macrophage and lymphocyte must share the same class II (Ia) antigen in order to have effective interaction.

12. The answer is A. *(IV B)* Immunologic tolerance can occur in an immunologically competent host when the host does not react to specific antigens produced by the graft. In such situations, the graft can survive almost indefinitely. In contrast to immunologic tolerance, immunologic enhancement involves antibodies on cells in the graft that block efficient antigen presentation by the graft.

13. The answer is C. *(IV A 3)* Chronic graft rejection may be due to specific antibody, sensitized cytotoxic T cells, or both. The antigens involved in this type of rejection are usually weak antigens not coded for by the HLA complex (antigens in minor histocompatibility loci). Rejection of the graft may be total or partial, with recovery of the graft.

14. The answer is D. [*II B 2 a (2)*] The β_2-microglobulin component of the class I HLA antigens is a nonpolymorphic protein of 12,000 daltons. It is not coded for in the HLA complex, which is controlled by a complex on chromosome 6, and is determined by a gene on chromosome 15. The entire molecule is anchored in the membrane by the alpha chain.

13
Tumor Immunology

I. INTRODUCTION

A. Definitions

1. **Neoplasms** result from new growth of cells (**neoplasia**) under conditions that would not ordinarily induce the multiplication of cells and, thus, the growth of tissue. Neoplasms are either benign or malignant.
   - **a. Benign neoplasms** are characterized by slow growth and restricted anatomic location, and do not usually cause death.
   - **b. Malignant neoplasms** are characterized by slow or rapid growth, anaplasia, invasion of the body, and metastases, and can result in death. Malignancies are termed **cancer**.

2. **Tumor** refers to the swelling resulting from neoplasia which is due primarily to an increase in tissue mass.

B. Evidence for an immune response to tumors. There is considerable evidence suggesting that the human body responds immunologically to tumors. This realization has its origin in the following clinical observations.

1. **Spontaneous regression** of human tumors (especially in malignant melanoma but also in neuroblastoma and other tumors) has been documented in over 100 published case reports.

2. Certain tumors demonstrate **long-term indolence**. That is, some tumors grow very slowly or seem to be quiescent until suddenly they metastasize and kill the patient.

3. The presence of a **mononuclear cellular response** in situ in inflammatory carcinomas correlates with improved survival rates. For example, persons with a breast carcinoma accompanied by an inflammatory response seem to do better than those with carcinomas that are not associated with inflammatory processes.

4. **After surgery it is common to detect malignant cells in the blood**; however, metastatic implantation is much more rare. Also one can demonstrate malignant cells in regional veins draining a tumor in one-third of the cases. However, this incidence is much higher than the number of people with metastatic tumors. In summary, metastatic cells are common, but the frequency of implantation and growth is low.

5. **Autologous tumors** fail to establish subcutaneously when malignant cells are transplanted from the tumor to such sites.

6. **Positive immediate and delayed hypersensitivity skin reaction tests** to autologous tumor cell extracts are readily demonstrated in cancer patients.

II. TUMOR-ASSOCIATED ANTIGENS. A distinct features of tumor immunology involves the interaction of the tumor-bearing host with a source of antigen that is constantly expanding. The quantity of tumor-associated antigen increases proportionally with tumor growth and decreases with tumor response to treatment.

A. General considerations

1. The progression from a normal cell to one with malignant potential is accompanied by many physiologic changes, such as dedifferentiation, acquisition of potential for perpetual reproduction (i.e., tumorigenesis, ability to form colonies in soft agar), loss of contact inhibition, and increased mitotic rate. In addition, the antigenic profile of the cells is altered such that normally occurring antigens may be lost while new epitopes emerge.

2. These neoantigens may be found in the nucleus, in the cytoplasm, or as a part of the cell membrane. Some are excreted from the cell.

   a. They may represent antigens completely unique to that particular tumor in that individual, but more commonly, they will be similar in all individuals carrying a particular tumor; such antigens are termed **tumor-specific antigens (TSAs)**. TSAs may be of **oncofetal** or **viral origin**.

   b. A subpopulation of TSAs can induce a protective immune response in the host. These are called **tumor-specific transplantation antigens (TSTAs)**.

   c. **Carcinogen-induced cancers** are often accompanied by the emergence of completely unique tumor-associated antigens. The carcinogen acts as a mutagen and the tumor induced by the same carcinogen will not have similar antigens, as is seen in malignancies of viral etiology, due to the random occurrence of the mutation.

B. Tumor-specific antigens (TSAs). It is perhaps a misnomer to consider any antigen as specific to a particular tumor type; however, there are antigens whose occurrence is highly correlated with certain tumors. These TSAs are not present in normal tissue cells but are found on the cell surface of tumors and elicit a specific immune response.

   1. Oncofetal antigens are present during normal fetal development but are lost during differentiation of fetal tissue, and their synthesis is not recognized during adult life. However, these antigens may reappear with the development of malignancy or during regeneration of the appropriate tissue (e.g., liver). Two of the most widely studied oncofetal antigens are alpha-fetoprotein and carcinoembryonic antigen (CEA).

   a. Alpha-fetoprotein is synthesized and secreted by fetal liver cells and can be detected in cord blood and, occasionally, in the mother's serum.

   (1) Most, but not all hepatomas (liver cancer) secrete large amounts of this alpha globulin. However, its presence is not diagnostic of hepatoma, but is merely suggestive. It has also been detected in the serum of patients with prostatic and gastric carcinomas, teratomas, and embryonal carcinoma of the testes.

   (2) Alpha-fetoprotein has been detected in nonmalignant conditions, such as cirrhosis of the liver and hepatitis.

   (3) By monitoring the changes in alpha-fetoprotein content of a patient's serum, a prognostic index (or **marker**) of surgical or chemotherapeutic success can be obtained. For example, a dramatic increase in the serum concentration would signal recurrence of the malignancy.

   b. CEA is detected in the gut, liver, and pancreas of normal human fetuses during the second trimester of pregnancy. It is found in low levels in the serum of normal adults.

   (1) High levels of CEA are present in the sera of about 70% of patients with carcinoma of the colon. An even higher association (90%) occurs in patients with pancreatic carcinoma. CEA has also been detected in significant quantities in cancers of the lung, breast, and prostate.

   (2) This antigen also occurs in nonmalignant states such as cigarette smoking (e.g., approximately 15% of heavy smokers will have elevated CEA levels in their serum), cirrhosis of the liver, and chronic lung disease.

   (3) As in the case of alpha-fetoprotein, the utility of CEA is in its prognostic potential.

   2. Another class of TSAs is of **viral origin**, being either **viral component proteins** or new **enzymes** induced in the cell to aid in the replication of the virus. These viral "fingerprints" form a major part of the evidence linking viruses with human malignancy; however, the etiologic role of viruses is more complex than this simple cause-and-effect relationship, because the same viruses that have been detected in human tumors are also found in noncancerous tissues. Antibodies to certain viral antigens have been found in the sera of tumor-bearing patients.

   a. Epstein-Barr virus (EBV) antigens have been found in the cells of patients with **Burkitt's lymphoma** and **nasopharyngeal carcinoma**. These patients have high levels of specific antibodies to EBV antigens, leading many investigators to speculate that Burkitt's lymphoma and nasopharyngeal carcinomas are induced by a viral agent.

   b. Other RNA and DNA viruses (e.g., the **adenovirus**, **papovavirus**, **herpesvirus**, and **leukemia–sarcoma viruses**) may also induce TSAs.

C. Tumor-specific transplantation antigens (TSTAs) occur on the membrane of the tumor cell. An appropriate immune response against these immunogens will favor control of the malignancy and elimination of the cancer cells from the body. As a general rule, the cell-mediated response is the most efficient tumoricidal mechanism, although, occasionally, cytocidal antibodies are also demonstrable in the host.

1. Most human tumors of a given histologic type will have at least one TSTA in common. Thus the lymphocytes and serum from neuroblastoma patient A will react with tumor cells from neuroblastoma patient B but not with other cells from the patient. They also will **not** react with tumor cells from patients suffering from other types of malignancies.

2. The realization that tumors are antigenic in the host and that the immune response against the tumor occurs very early in tumorigenesis led to development of the concept of **immune surveillance**. By this mechanism, the body is continuously purging itself of potentially cancerous cells, which probably arise frequently during a person's life span. Thus, cancer is an escape or bypass of this protective mechanism; factors that decrease immune capabilities predispose an individual to malignancy.

III. IMMUNE RESPONSE TO TUMOR ANTIGENS. The interaction between the host and tumor that it harbors is extremely complex (Fig. 13-1). The immune response attempts to rid the body of the tumor cells (now recognized as foreign because they have acquired new antigens). However, the tumor produces soluble antigens, which tend to neutralize these protective responses. In addition, some humoral antibodies may actually enhance tumor growth. The eventual outcome of the encounter is determined by factors that are poorly understood.

  A. Protective responses. TSTA-specific sensitized lymphocytes constitute the major immunologic barrier against cancer. In addition, specific antibodies may help rid the body of tumor cells. They may act in a complement-dependent cytolytic manner or may function by "arming" lymphocytes or macrophages of the body such that these cells can then react with and destroy tumor cells.

  B. Mechanisms of tumor rejection. Both specific and nonspecific immune responses—humoral and cell-mediated—are believed to be involved in the rejection of a tumor.

    1. **T cells** play the dominant role in defending the body against tumor growth. The cytocidal effects of these cells are stimulated by antigens (see Chapter 5, section V B 2 d) such as TSAs or viral antigens. **Cytotoxic T (Tc) cells** appear in response to TSAs and can kill the tumor cells by direct contact. The membrane marker for Tc cells is the T8 antigen.

    2. **B-cell involvement** is manifested by antibody formation. The antibody that is formed can react with a tumor cell; however, both experimental models and studies in humans demonstrate that antibody is not very effective in causing tumor rejection, particularly solid tumors. Antibody may play some role in the control of leukemia. Passive administration of antibody to which toxins such as ricin have been conjugated, hold some promise in the immunotherapy of malignancy.

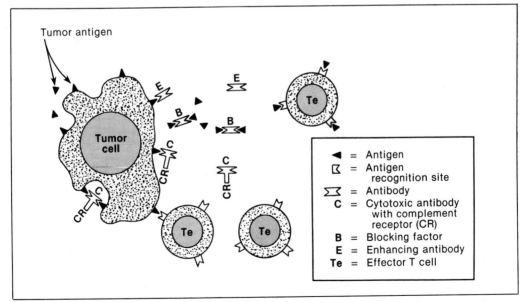

Figure 13-1. Potential host immune responses to tumors: those at the top half of the cell favor tumor growth; those at the bottom are cytotoxic.

    a. Killer (K) cells (non-T, non-B, null cells) have an Fc receptor on their membrane. If they encounter a tumor cell that has IgG molecules on its surface they will interact with that "sensitized" cell and destroy it. This process is called **antibody-dependent cellular cytotoxicity (ADCC)**. The K cell does the killing; the process is independent of complement and requires much less antibody (i.e., several hundred-fold) than does antibody-dependent complement lysis.

    b. Complement-dependent cytotoxicity can also be mediated by antibodies, particularly IgM. As antibody binds to the surface of the tumor cell, the **classical complement pathway** (see Chapter 4, section II A 2) is triggered, leading to the eventual destruction of the tumor cell.

3. Natural killer (NK) cells (non-T, non-B cells) are present without the host ever being exposed to tumors.

    a. NK cells recognize malignant cells but not normal cells. The tumor cells are killed via a direct interaction between the NK cells and the tumor cells (by the same mechanism as Tc cells). NK cells also have Fc receptors; however, these cells can kill without any attached antibody.

    b. Morphologically, NK cells also are associated with **large granular lymphocytes (LGL)**. It is believed that NK cells are responsible for **immune surveillance**, the theory holding that malignant transformations occur continually. The NK cells may be responsible for preventing these transformations from being expressed.

4. Macrophages in their normal state are not very cytotoxic. However, they can kill tumor cells when activated.

    a. Antibodies to TSAs may simultaneously bind to tumor cells and macrophages, thus forming a bridge that activates **macrophage-mediated cytotoxicity** leading to tumor cell death.

    b. In vivo sensitized T cells are triggered to release a lymphokine called **macrophage-activating factor (MAF)**. The MAF interacts with macrophages, changes their metabolism, and makes them potent killers of tumor cells. Activated macrophages do not rely on interacting with any specific tumor antigen, but, like NK cells, do seem to distinguish malignant from normal cells.

    c. Because activated macrophages are such potent killers, there is much interest at the clinical level in treating people with compounds known to activate macrophages [e.g., bacille Calmette-Guerin (BCG, the mycobacterial vaccine used to immunize against tuberculosis); *Corynebacterium parvum*; and **muramyl dipeptide**, a small peptide molecule that can be extracted from any mycobacterium].

    d. Antitumor products of macrophages include:

      (1) Hydrolytic enzymes which degrade connective tissue and activate several humoral mediators (e.g., complement components and coagulation factors)

      (2) Interferon, which has indirect action due to activation of NK cells

      (3) Tumor necrosis factor (TNF), also known as **cachectin**, a protein which induces other cells to release interleukin-1 and beta-interferon

      (4) Oxidative products [e.g., hydrogen peroxide (see Chapter 1, section II C 3)] of the glycolysis that accompanies phagocytosis, which can be directly toxic to tumor cells by perturbating the cell membrane

      (5) Complement components and factors B, D, and P of the alternative pathway, which can play a role in tumor cell lysis and also act as chemotaxins (see Chapter 4, section II B 2)

C. Immunotherapeutic principles of treating human tumors include the following.

  1. Reduction of tumor "load" by surgery, or chemotherapy, or both

  2. Modification of tumor cells to enhance antigenicity and eliminate viability

  3. Activation of the immune response via adjuvants

D. Immunologic factors favoring tumor growth

  1. Immune enhancement occurs when specific antibodies in the serum protect tumor cells from cell-mediated destruction.

    a. Immunostimulation of tumor growth may occur due to low numbers of Tc cells.

    b. Blocking factors also have been suggested as enhancers of tumor growth. The serum of patients often contains soluble TSTA or TSTA–antibody complexes, which react with the tumor-specific receptors on sensitized T cells and prevent their cytotoxic interaction with tumor cells.

    c. Tumor growth enhancers include the following.

      (1) Free soluble tumor antigen interacts with the tumor antigen recognition site on the lymphocyte surface. This triggers the activity of the lymphocyte but it can cause a problem if the lymphocyte is triggered at a site away from the solid tumor as the lymphokines (e.g. lymphotoxin) will not have an opportunity to act on the tumor cell. Free tumor antigen also could mask the tumor antigen recognition site and actually not trigger the lymphocyte, which would prevent the T cell from recognizing and attacking the tumor cell.

   (2) Modulation of tumor antigenicity (antigenic modulation) occurs when antibody to the tumor cell reacts with the appropriate antigens on the tumor cell surface. If the antibody is cytotoxic, tumor cells expressing the homologous antigen will be destroyed, favoring the emergence of tumor cells that have a different membrane antigenic mosaic.

   (3) Antigen–antibody complexes act like free tumor antigen and mask the tumor recognition sites of T cells, thus preventing the T cells from recognizing and attacking the tumor cells. It paralyzes the T cells in a state of nonreactivity. The most potent serum blocking factors are the tumor-specific immune complexes that appear in the body.

2. Suppressor cells serve as another mechanism promoting tumor growth.
   a. Suppressor T (Ts) cells (with T8 membrane marker). For some reason, tumor antigens are more conducive to the activation of Ts cells than Tc cells. Ts cells can interact with Tc cells and eliminate their reactivity, thus down-regulating the immune response. They are abundant in tumor patients and suppress the immune response to the point where it becomes ineffective in eliminating the tumor.
   b. Suppressor macrophages are poorly characterized but, like Ts cells, they appear to depress the T-cell system. Certain immunostimulants (e.g., BCG and *C. parvum*) have been found to intensify macrophage-mediated suppression.

3. Immune selection
   a. The immune response to tumor cells will eliminate those cells with the strongest antigen but will not be as effective on cells with lesser concentrations of antigen or with weaker antigens. Thus, the most antigenic cells will be killed off and the least antigenic will survive.
   b. In certain cases, metastatic tumors will lack antigen, allowing a phenomenon termed "sneaking through" to occur. In its initial growth, the tumor only contains a few cells. The immune response to these cells is very small and somehow lags behind the responses necessary to kill the cells. As more cells appear, the immune response is still deficient and is never able to overcome and control the malignancy.

4. Ontogenetic status. At certain times of life, the immune response is poorly developed or very weak. This is especially true in the neonatal period and in old age. Indeed, at these extremes the incidence of malignancy is highest.

5. Immunologic deficiency may be hereditary or may be induced via such means as irradiation or immunosuppressive drugs. The incidence of malignancy is greatly increased in such individuals.

6. Tumor cell attributes often allow the tumor to escape destruction.
   a. Rapid tumor growth allows it to outstrip the immune response which is weak and slow by comparison.
   b. Tumors release immunosuppressive factors such as alpha-fetoprotein and prostaglandins. Many of the tumor-inducing viruses studied in animal models are immunosuppressive.
   c. Tumor heterogeneity allows tumor survival more substantially than any other factor.
      (1) During growth, a tumor can change its antigens, its metastatic potential, or virtually any attribute of tumor biology that can be measured.
      (2) Part of the reason for the change in antigens is the antigenic modulation phenomenon [see section III D 1 c (2)], but, in addition, the tumor can simply change its antigenic makeup genetically. Tumor heterogeneity allows the tumor to escape immune destruction.

IV. NEUROBLASTOMA MODEL. Neuroblastoma, a malignancy that begins development in utero and expresses itself early in the life of the infant, has been a convenient model for the study of the immune responses of humans to their tumors. Observations which have been made in this tumor–host system are listed here to summarize and exemplify our understanding of this complex relationship.

A. The lymphocytes of children with neuroblastoma are cytotoxic to these tumor cells but express no toxicity against normal cells or cells of other tumors.

B. The lymphocytes from mothers of children with neuroblastoma demonstrate in vitro tumor-specific cytotoxicity toward neuroblastoma tumor cells but not other types of tumor cells.

C. In some situations, both the child and the mother have antibodies that are cytotoxic for the neuroblastoma cells. In other cases of neuroblastoma, the serum does not kill the tumor cells but rather protects them via blocking factors such as antigen–antibody complexes. These relationships are presented graphically in Figure 13-2.

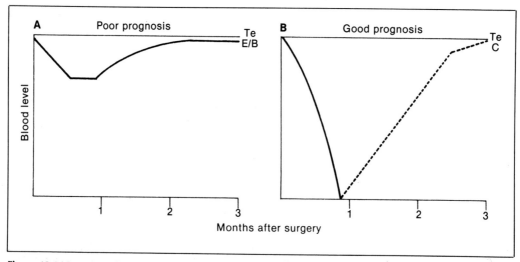

Figure 13-2. Presence of tumor enhancing (A) and tumoricidal (B) factors in the blood as a function of time after surgical removal of the tumor mass. *Te* = effector T cell; *E/B* = enhancing/blocking factors; *C* = cytotoxic antibody.

STUDY QUESTIONS

Directions: Each question below contains five suggested answers. Choose the **one best** response to each question.

1. The strongest evidence for the role of the immune system in preventing the establishment of tumors (immune surveillance) is

(A) the hereditary pattern of malignancies
(B) the peak incidence of malignancies in the age group 10 to 40 years
(C) the rapid transformation of normal cells to malignant cells in vitro where the immune system is not available
(D) the markedly increased incidence of malignancies in persons with congenital or acquired immune deficiencies
(E) the paucity of tumors in the very young

2. When viruses transform cells and cause tumors, new antigens appear in the cells. Which one of the following statements is uniformly true about these antigens?

(A) These antigens are found in the plasma membrane, cytoplasm, nucleus, or all of these locations
(B) These antigens are oncofetal antigens
(C) These antigens are tumor-specific transplantation antigens (TSTAs)
(D) These antigens will be a component of the mature virus
(E) These antigens will be unique to that tumor in that host

3. A unique (individualistic) tumor-specific antigen (TSA) found in only a single tumor and not present in any other tumor, whether of the same or different histologic type, can best be explained by

(A) a viral etiology
(B) derepression of the expression of a fetal antigen
(C) a random mutational event
(D) immunosuppression of the host
(E) faulty immune surveillence of the host

4. All of the following are naturally occurring components of the immune response to malignancies EXCEPT

(A) a heightened general immune responsiveness
(B) specific cellular immunity via lymphocytes
(C) cytotoxic antibodies that destroy tumor cells
(D) enhancing antibodies that interfere with the immunologic attack on tumor cells
(E) modulation of tumor antigenicity

Directions: Each question below contains four suggested answers of which **one or more** is correct. Choose the answer

A   if **1, 2, and 3** are correct
B   if **1 and 3** are correct
C   if **2 and 4** are correct
D   if **4** is correct
E   if **1, 2, 3, and 4** are correct

5. Immunosuppressive factors secreted by tumor cells include

(1) antibodies
(2) prostaglandins
(3) muramyl dipeptide
(4) tumor-specific transplantation antigens (TSTAs)

6. Human malignancies associated with tumor-specific antigens (TSAs) include

(1) carcinoma of the colon
(2) neuroblastoma
(3) hepatoma
(4) Burkitt's lymphoma

SUMMARY OF DIRECTIONS

A	B	C	D	E
1, 2, 3 only	1, 3 only	2, 4 only	4 only	All are correct

---

7. Immunologic factors favoring tumor growth

(1) may act by binding to tumor cells and protecting the cells from cytotoxic lymphocytes
(2) may be composed of tumor-specific transplantation antigen (TSTA)–antibody complexes
(3) may act by binding to immune lymphocytes and neutralizing their action against tumor cells
(4) may cause a change in the antigenic composition of the tumor

8. Oncofetal antigens are tumor-specific antigens (TSAs) that are

(1) normal components of embryonic and regenerating tissues
(2) prognostic indicators used to follow patients undergoing therapy for certain malignancies
(3) found as membrane components or may be secreted from cells
(4) diagnostic of malignancy

9. Prevention of, and recovery from, cancer may involve

(1) natural killer (NK) cells
(2) macrophages
(3) killer (K) cells
(4) suppressor T (Ts) cells

10. Immune responses favoring tumor growth include

(1) immunologic anergy
(2) blocking factors
(3) enhancing antibodies
(4) cellular immunity

11. Cellular changes associated with the progression from normal to malignant include

(1) increased mitotic rate
(2) acquisition of new membrane antigens
(3) loss of contact inhibition
(4) loss of membrane antigens

12. Neuroblastoma is a malignancy that occurs predominantly in infants. Facts about the host response to neuroblastoma which suggest protective immune responses to malignancy include

(1) patient lymphocytes are cytotoxic for neuroblastoma cells
(2) patient lymphocytes are cytotoxic for other tumor cells (e.g., melanoma)
(3) mothers of patients commonly have lymphocytes that are cytotoxic for neuroblastoma cells
(4) serum of patient protects tumor cells from cytotoxic lymphocytes

ANSWERS AND EXPLANATIONS

1. The answer is D. (*III D 4, 5, 6*) Immune depression, either congenital or induced by chemotherapy, is associated with a high incidence of infections and malignancies. Very young (neonate) and aged individuals also have an elevated incidence of cancer (when compared to individuals in the 10- to 50-year-old age group), and these people also are somewhat immunologically deficient.

2. The answer is A. (*II A 2*) Virally induced neoantigens can occur any place in the host cell. They are not oncofetal antigens in that they do not occur normally during fetal development. Some will be transplantation antigens, but those which occur inside the cell cannot play a role in tumor rejection. Most will be components of the virus, but some may be early proteins used in viral synthesis and/or assembly. Antigens induced by chemical carcinogens are unique to each tumor as they are the result of a specific mutation. The immunologic specificity of tumor antigens induced by viruses is controlled by the virus, hence they will be identical if the virus is the same, regardless of the host (or tumor).

3. The answer is C. (*II A 2 c*) A random mutation would result in a completely unique tumor-specific antigen (TSA). Virally induced tumors share antigens. Derepression of a gene which codes for a protein produced during fetal development would not lead to a unique antigen. Immune surveillence controls the expression of malignant potential; it does not control the immunologic specificity of the tumor.

4. The answer is A. [*III A, B 1, 2 b, D 1 b*] As a rule, the development of malignancy is accompanied by a decrease in the immune responsiveness of the individual. In fact, immunosuppression favors the development of tumors, as evidenced by the increased incidence of cancer in transplant recipients and patients with immunodeficiency diseases.

5. The answer is C (2, 4). (*III D 1 b, 6 b*) Tumor-specific transplantation antigens (TSTAs) can interfere with the protective action of cytotoxic cells and complement-fixing antibodies. Prostaglandins are secreted by certain tumors and exert a general immunosuppressive action. Antibodies are secreted by plasma cells, not tumor cells. Muramyl dipeptide is an immunoaugmentor found in the cell wall of many bacteria (especially active in mycobacteria) which enhances macrophage activity.

6. The answer is E (all). [*II B 1 a, b, 2 a, c (1)*] Tumor-specific antigens (TSAs) are found on the cell surface of particular tumors. Carcinoembryonic antigen (CEA) is an oncofetal antigen associated with carcinoma of the colon and pancreas. Alpha-fetoprotein is another oncofetal antigen; it is found in fetal tissues and in the serum of most patients with primary carcinoma of the liver (hepatoma). It is also associated with prostatic carcinoma, other malignancies, hepatitis and cirrhosis of the liver. The patients with neuroblastoma usually have lymphocytes which are specifically cytotoxic for cells from their own and histologically similar tumors. This fact implies that these tumors also have specific antigens, in this particular case, a tumor-specific transplantation antigen (TSTA). Patients with Burkitt's lymphoma have high levels of specific antibodies to Epstein-Barr virus (EBV) antigen, leading many investigators to speculate about the viral origin of this malignant neoplasm.

7. The answer is E (all). (*III D 1, 3*) Factors favoring tumor growth can readily be demonstrated in vitro and, unfortunately, are usually effective in vivo as well. They may "coat" tumor-specific transplantation antigens (TSTAs) and interfere with the antitumor effects of cytotoxic cells such as lymphocytes and macrophages. Similarly, they may compete with complement-fixing antibodies for TSTAs on the cell membrane. If these blocking factors react with cytotoxic cells at a site distant from the tumor, the antitumor action of these cells may be dissipated before it can exert a protective effect.

8. The answer is A (1, 2, 3). (*II B 1*) Oncofetal antigens are normal components of developing tissues which may be excreted or many be components of the cell itself. Their value is as a prognostic indicator of the potential for relapse (i.e., the efficacy of surgical or other therapeutic intervention). These antigens are induced by so many diverse factors (e.g., cigarette smoking) that their use in diagnosis is contraindicated; the number of false-positives is too great.

9. The answer is A (1, 2, 3). (*III B 2 a, 3, 4, D 2 a*) Natural killer (NK) cells are responsible for the control of spontaneous mutations that occur which could result in malignancy. Like the macrophage and the killer (K) cell, NK cells are immune surveillence mechanisms of the body that are present in the absence of antigenic exposure. K cell function requires antibody "arming" [these are the cells of antibody-dependent cellular cytoxicity (ADCC)], and macrophage antitumor function is enhanced by antibody. Suppressor cells serve to down-regulate the immune response and would enhance tumor growth.

10. The answer is A (1, 2, 3). (*III B 1, D 1, 2*) Enhancing (non-complement–fixing) antibodies and blocking factors [tumor-specific transplantation antigen (TSTA) or TSTA–antibody complexes] favor tumor growth as does immunologic anergy (a general depression of immune responsiveness of the individual). Intact cellular immunity, as expressed by competent cytotoxic lymphocyte development, acts to control tumor development, as do activated macrophages and cytotoxic (complement-fixing) antibodies.

11. The answer is E (all). [*II A 1, 2; III D 1 (2)*] Malignant cells are usually dedifferentiated, have potential for uncontrolled growth (i.e., they are immortal), and do not express growth inhibition when they come in contact with other similar cells. They usually acquire new epitopes not uncommonly at the expense of preexisting differentiated antigens.

12. The answer is B (1, 3). (*IV A, B, D*) Neuroblastoma is a malignancy of early infancy and early childhood. The lymphocytes of the patients (and, sometimes, their mothers) kill neuroblastoma cells but not cells from other malignancies. The serum of the patient may contain enhancing factors such as noncomplement-fixing antibodies or antigen–antibody complexes, or it may contain antibodies involved in cytotoxicity or the antibody-dependent cellular cytotoxic (ADCC) reaction.

Post-test

QUESTIONS

Directions: Each question below contains five suggested answers. Choose the **one best** response to each question.

1. The rapid rise, elevated level, and prolonged production of antibody that follows a second exposure to antigen is known as

(A) delayed hypersensitivity reaction
(B) autoimmune response
(C) anamnestic response
(D) conditioned response
(E) thymus-independent response

2. What is the most direct method of treating atopic allergies?

(A) Hyposensitization
(B) Environmental control
(C) Administration of modified allergens
(D) Antihistamines
(E) Corticosteroids

3. The mechanism of immunologic rejection of normal tissue transplants is similar to that seen in tumor rejection. The mechanism that is unique to tumor rejection is produced by

(A) natural killer (NK) cells
(B) antibody and complement
(C) cytotoxic T (Tc) cells
(D) antibody and macrophages
(E) antibody and killer (K) cells

4. Theoretically, each of the following goals should be attempted in the immunotherapy of cancer EXCEPT

(A) reduction of the tumor burden to the lowest possible level by surgery, drugs, or irradiation
(B) use of soluble tumor antigens to stimulate antibodies
(C) activation of macrophages and lymphocytes by adjuvants such as bacille Calmette-Guérin and *Corynebacterium parvum*
(D) use of viable tumor cells for specific immunization of the patient
(E) bolstering immune function with substances such as interferon and interleukin-2

5. The sites in or on antigens with which antibodies react are called

(A) haplotypes
(B) isotopes
(C) isotypes
(D) epitopes
(E) idiotypes

6. Antibodies may inhibit an immune response by all of the following mechanisms EXCEPT

(A) killing B cells
(B) killing T cells
(C) killing macrophages
(D) killing neutrophils
(E) binding antigen and preventing its access to antibody-forming tissues

↳ not antigen processing cells so
no role in immune response. **153**

7. All of the following cells experience major histocompatibility (MHC) restriction EXCEPT

(A) helper T (Th) cells
(B) B cells
(C) macrophages
(D) suppressor T (Ts) cells
(E) natural killer (NK) cells

8. The binding site for complement on the IgG immunoglobulin molecule is in the

(A) V_L domain
(B) C_L domain
(C) V_H domain
(D) C_H1 domain
(E) C_H2 domain

9. True statements concerning histocompatibility antigens include which of the following?

(A) They are composed of nucleic acids
(B) They are controlled solely by genes on autosomal chromosomes
(C) They do not induce a graft-versus-host (GVH) reaction
(D) They are located at the cell surface
(E) In humans, they are found in a segment of chromosome 17

10. The capacity of a molecule to react specifically with a product of induced lymphoid cell differentiation is known as

(A) antigenic specificity
(B) antigenicity
(C) affinity
(D) avidity
(E) immunogenicity

11. All of the following are macrophage properties, EXCEPT the presence in the membrane of

(A) IgE Fc receptors
(B) IgG Fc receptors
(C) C3b receptors
(D) Ia antigens
(E) IgM Fc receptors

12. Unique amino acid sequences located in the variable (V) region of immunoglobulin molecules and associated with the antigen-binding capability of the molecule are called

(A) allotypes
(B) subclasses
(C) idiotypes
(D) domains
(E) isotypes

13. The most important antigenic system that must be evaluated for organ allotransplantation in humans is

(A) Rh
(B) ABO
(C) Gm
(D) HLA
(E) H-2

14. RhoGAM is used in human medicine to prevent

(A) erythroblastosis fetalis
(B) transfusion reactions
(C) hepatitis A in an exposed individual
(D) hepatitis B in an exposed individual
(E) graft-versus-host (GVH) disease in the recipient of a bone marrow transplant

15. Examples of specific immune globulin (SIG) serum preparations include all of the following EXCEPT

(A) rabies immune globulin
(B) hepatitis A immune globulin
(C) hepatitis B immune globulin
(D) varicella zoster immune globulin
(E) Rh immune globulin

16. Initial laboratory workup of an immunodeficient patient reveals a positive mumps skin test, a positive Schick test (an inflammatory reaction at the site of diphtheria toxin injection), adequate chemotactic and intracellular killing activities, and serum that caused the hemolysis of antibody sensitized erythrocytes. The child most likely has a defect in

(A) T cells
(B) B cells
(C) T cells and B cells
(D) complement
(E) phagocytes

Question 17

Pictured below is an Ouchterlony plate.

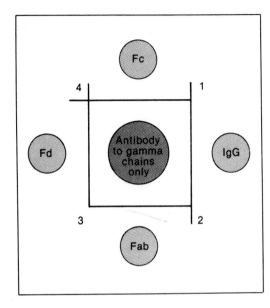

17. Concerning the elements shown in the Ouchterlony plate above, all of the following statements are true EXCEPT

(A) there is a spur at (1) because antibody to V_H and C_H1 domains will not react with Fc
(B) the antibody in spur (2) is specific for C_H2 and C_H3 domains
(C) the line of identity at (3) forms because Fd is a part of Fab
(D) the lines of nonidentity at (4) form because Fc = C_H2 and C_H3 domains while Fd = V_H and C_H1 domains
(E) the precipitin pattern would be the same if the center well contained antibody specific for light chains

18. The delicate balance between effective chemotherapy and iatrogenic (physician-induced) disease is well exemplified in the case of the treatment of human malignancies, where many of the therapeutic agents used to arrest the growth of the cancer cells will also cause

(A) hepatotoxic manifestations
(B) aplastic anemia
(C) immunosuppression
(D) drug allergies
(E) autoimmune diseases

19. Recurrent pyogenic infections, defective processing of polysaccharide antigens, a T-cell deficit, elevated levels of IgA and IgE, and depressed levels of IgM are characteristics of

(A) acquired immune deficiency syndrome (AIDS)
(B) chronic mucocutaneous candidiasis
(C) severe combined immunodeficiency (SCID)
(D) common variable hypogammaglobulinemia
(E) Wiskott-Aldrich syndrome

20. The major antibody in immune globulin (IG) is

(A) IgA
(B) IgD
(C) IgE
(D) IgG
(E) IgM

21. In transfusion reactions that occur due to extravascular hemolysis of red blood cells, the hemolytic reaction almost invariably involves

(A) IgE
(B) complement
(C) anti-A antibodies
(D) anti-B antibodies
(E) anti-Rh antibodies

22. Specific immunologic tolerance is most easily induced in

(A) T cells
(B) B cells
(C) macrophages
(D) T cells and B cells, which are equally sensitive
(E) T cells, B cells, and macrophages, which are equally sensitive

23. The pathogenetic mechanism of tissue injury in cytotoxic (type II) reactions is initiated by

(A) antibody interfering with the functioning of biologically active substances
(B) antigen reacting with cell-bound antibody
(C) antibody reacting with cell-bound antigen
(D) formation of antigen–antibody complexes
(E) antigen-reactive T cells reacting with specific antigens

Questions 24 and 25

An 18-year-old woman from a socially deprived background is admitted to the hospital in labor. On admission, she indicates that her pregnancy has been apparently normal despite receiving essentially no prenatal care. However, she admits to having been sexually promiscuous but denies the occurrence of a lesion suggestive of syphilis. Shortly after admission, she gives birth to an apparently healthy male infant.

24. At delivery, the procedure of choice used to determine the presence of venereal disease in the mother is

(A) Coombs (antiglobulin) test
(B) flocculation
(C) toxin–antitoxin reaction
(D) lysis
(E) precipitation

25. The mother's serum was positive for a diagnosis of syphilis. Although the infant remained asymptomatic, it was decided to monitor him carefully for possible signs of congenital syphilis by testing his serum levels of

(A) IgA
(B) IgD
(C) IgE
(D) IgG
(E) IgM

Directions: Each question below contains four suggested answers of which **one or more** is correct. Choose the answer

A if **1, 2, and 3** are correct
B if **1 and 3** are correct
C if **2 and 4** are correct
D if **4** is correct
E if **1, 2, 3, and 4** are correct

26. Chronic granulomatous disease is characterized by

(1) recurrent bacterial infections
(2) hepatosplenomegaly
(3) defective oxidative burst by neutrophils
(4) reduction in intracellular reduced nicotinamide adenine dinucleotide (NADH) level

27. Humoral nonantibody factors contributing to natural immunity include

(1) lymphokine activated killer (LAK) cells
(2) beta lysin
(3) bacteriolysis
(4) properdin

28. Immune response (Ir) genes can be described as

(1) being associated with the major histocompatibility complex (MHC)
(2) specifying the ability of an animal to recognize and respond to certain antigens
(3) exerting their control through T lymphocytes
(4) being ultimately expressed as immunoglobulin formation

29. Mediators of immediate hypersensitivity (type I) reactions are classified either as preformed in mediator cells or as newly formed constituents released after initiation of the reaction. Preformed mediators of type I reactions include

(1) platelet-activating factor (PAF)
(2) eosinophil chemotactic factor of anaphylaxis (ECF-A)
(3) slow-reacting substance of anaphylaxis (SRS-A)
(4) serotonin (5-hydroxytryptamine)

30. In the induction of delayed hypersensitivity, interaction between antigen-processing cells and T cells can only occur if the two participants

(1) possess Km markers
(2) are idiotype-identical
(3) possess identical class I antigens
(4) are major histocompatibility complex (MHC)-identical

31. A preparation of pooled human IgM injected into a rabbit may stimulate production of antibodies reactive with

(1) $\varkappa$ chain
(2) μ chain
(3) λ chain
(4) J chain

Questions 32–34

A 54-year-old pathologist was in good health until 12 days prior to hospital admission when, after receiving an influenza vaccination, he developed generalized malaise. The condition persisted for 6 days, and he became concerned that it was more than a mere vaccination reaction. Four days prior to admission he developed a severe headache with accompanying bone and muscle pain. Two days prior to admission he developed weakness of the extremities. On the day of admission he had been unable to get out of bed and was brought to the hospital by ambulance.

Physical examination revealed a well-developed, well-nourished, white male in moderate respiratory distress with rapid, shallow breathing. Blood pressure was 160/120, pulse 86, and respirations 32/min. The remainder of the physical examination was unremarkable, except for the muscular weakness and slight neurologic impairment. A lumbar puncture was performed and revealed the following: Opening pressure—normal; appearance—clear; sugar—60 mg/dl; chloride—120 mEq/L; leukocytes—absent; erythrocytes—3–4 per high-power field; protein—39 mg/dl. During the next 2 days, the patient's pulmonary capacity decreased from 3600 ml to 1000 ml. Blood gases at this time were P_{O_2}, 70, and P_{CO_2}, 48, with a pH of 7.41. A tracheostomy was performed, and the patient was placed on a respirator.

During the next 4 weeks, the patient's condition continued to deteriorate. His paralysis became almost complete. He developed pneumococcal pneumonia, which was treated successfully with penicillin. Seven weeks after admission he began to regain neurologic function. His muscular strength returned slowly, and his pulmonary function improved such that the respirator was discontinued on the sixty-third hospital day. He was discharged 2 weeks later and placed on an active physical therapy program. Recovery was complete, and 6 months after his initial illness the patient was able to return to work full-time.

32. The patient's symptoms were originally muscular and then became neurologic. Autoimmune diseases that would affect these tissues include

(1) systemic lupus erythematosus (SLE)
(2) multiple sclerosis
(3) myasthenia gravis
(4) Guillain-Barré syndrome

33. What immunologic tests could be performed to confirm or exclude each of these potential diagnoses?

(1) Systemic lupus erythematosus (SLE)—indirect immunofluorescence to detect antinuclear antibodies
(2) Multiple sclerosis—spinal fluid IgG testing
(3) Myasthenia gravis—acetylcholine receptor antibodies
(4) Guillain-Barré syndrome—complement fixation test

34. The life-threatening component of the man's symptomatology was pulmonary embarrassment. Why was a lumbar puncture performed?

(1) To rule out a brain abscess
(2) To aid in administration of antibiotics
(3) To confirm suspicion of increased intracranial pressure
(4) To rule out encephalomyelitis

Question 35

The director of the hospital radioimmunoassay laboratory needs an antiserum that will react specifically with gentamicin. He suggests the following protocol for production of the antiserum:

- intramuscular injection of a rabbit with 5 mg of gentamicin dissolved in sterile physiologic saline
- repetition of the injection 10 days later
- bleeding the rabbit 10 days after the second injection
- repetition of the three procedures listed above until a satisfactory immune response is obtained

35. The immunologist's recommendation should include

(1) chemically conjugating the antibiotic to a carrier molecule before injection
(2) utilizing human erythrocytes as the test vehicle
(3) increasing the number of animals
(4) adjusting the route of administration and the dosage of the antibiotic

36. Immune complexes in serum and other biological fluids can be detected by the

(1) Prausnitz-Küstner (PK) reaction
(2) Raji cell binding assay
(3) radioallergosorbent (RAST) test
(4) C1q binding assay

SUMMARY OF DIRECTIONS

A	B	C	D	E
1, 2, 3 only	1, 3 only	2, 4 only	4 only	All are correct

Questions 37 and 38

A 52-year-old man presents with the complaint of blood in his stools. He reports that he has experienced some changes in his bowel habits over the last 1½ years and recently has become aware of the sensation that his evacuations are not complete. Proctoscopic examination reveals a large ulcerating mass in the descending colon. Biopsy results confirm the diagnosis of carcinoma of the colon, and the malignant mass is surgically removed. The patient is placed on appropriate chemotherapy and discharged 2 weeks later to be followed in the oncology clinic. Monthly blood specimens taken during the next year reveal the following carcinoembryonic antigen (CEA) levels:

	CEA (ng/ml)
Preoperative sample	50
Postoperative sample (day 1)	65
Month 1	15
Month 2	5
Months 3–9	< 2.5
Month 10	10
Month 11	25
Month 12	40

37. Clinically, the performance of assays for CEA levels was considered to be of significance due to the usefulness of CEA in

(1) localization of certain tumors in vivo
(2) diagnosing carcinoma of the colon
(3) diagnosing carcinoma of the pancreas
(4) follow-up for the recurrence of certain malignancies

38. The CEA levels obtained during months 10–12 for this patient indicate

(1) the development of metastases
(2) the initial diagnosis of carcinoma of the colon was incorrect
(3) surgical removal of the tumor was incomplete
(4) a revised diagnosis of carcinoma of the pancreas is warranted

Questions 39 and 40

A Boy Scout troop in New Jersey is planning a summer trip to a remote region of Colorado. As a precaution, the boys receive booster shots for tetanus and typhoid fever. One week later, blood samples are drawn to determine whether the boys are responding to the vaccines.

39. Serologic tests that could be used to detect antibodies to the tetanus toxin include

(1) toxin neutralization
(2) complement fixation
(3) precipitation
(4) agglutination

40. Serologic tests that could be used to detect antibodies to the typhoid bacillus include

(1) bacterial agglutination
(2) bactericidal assay
(3) complement fixation
(4) indirect immunofluorescence

Questions 41–43

An acutely ill 2-year-old boy is brought to the emergency room. His breathing is extremely labored, and he is producing rust-colored sputum. A Gram stain of the sputum reveals numerous gram-positive cocci in random clusters. A diagnosis of staphylococcal pneumonia is made, and the child is hospitalized and placed on intravenous methicillin. It is disclosed that the child had experienced several such episodes previously that had been successfully controlled with antibiotics. Further discussion of the child's medical history reveals that he had experienced a normal recovery from measles, approximately 6 months earlier.

41. This revelation excludes certain diseases from the differential diagnosis including

(1) DiGeorge syndrome
(2) Nezelof's syndrome
(3) Wiskott-Aldrich syndrome
(4) selective immunoglobulin deficiency

Leukocyte function studies are performed and indicate that phagocytosis, intracellular killing, and chemotactic responses are all within normal limits.

42. These features rule out defects in nonspecific resistance, such as

(1) chronic granulomatous disease
(2) lazy leukocyte syndrome
(3) Job's syndrome
(4) de Vaal syndrome

An immunoglobulin profile is ordered. The child has no detectable immunoglobulin A (IgA) or IgM in his serum. A small amount (30 mg/dl) of IgG is detected when the assay is repeated with low level radial immunodiffusion plates.

43. Based on this information, possible diagnoses include

(1) selective immunoglobulin deficiency
(2) common variable hypogammaglobulinemia
(3) Wiskott-Aldrich syndrome
(4) Bruton's hypogammaglobulinemia

Directions: For each numbered item below, select the one lettered choice with which it is most closely associated. Each lettered choice may be used once, more than once, or not at all. Choose the answer

    A if the item is associated with **(A) only**
    B if the item is associated with **(B) only**
    C if the item is associated with **both (A) and (B)**
    D if the item is associated with **neither (A) nor (B)**

Questions 44–47

Match each characteristic to the cell with which it is most frequently associated.

(A) B cell
(B) T cell
(C) Both
(D) Neither

44. IgM and IgD in membrane

45. C3b receptor contained on membrane

46. Principally involved in graft rejection

47. Interaction with a macrophage has class II antigen restriction

48. Hyperacute graft rejection may be caused by

(A) blood group incompatibility between donor and recipient
(B) previous sensitization of female recipients as a result of multiparity
(C) both
(D) neither

49. The plasma of a healthy person that is blood group AB will demonstrate which isohemagglutinin?

(A) anti-A isohemagglutinin
(B) anti-B isohemagglutinin
(C) both
(D) neither

Directions: The groups of questions below consist of lettered choices followed by several numbered items. For each numbered item select the **one** lettered choice with which it is **most** closely associated. Each lettered choice may be used once, more than once, or not at all.

Questions 50–53

For each characteristic, select the immunoglobulin associated with it.

(A) IgD
(B) IgA
(C) IgE
(D) IgG
(E) IgM

D 50. Fixes complement efficiently via the C_H2 domain

E 51. Fixation occurs via the C_H4 domain

B 52. Fixes complement via the alternative pathway only

E 53. Fixes complement most efficiently of all the immunoglobulins

Questions 54–56

Match each description of laboratory techniques below with the technique it best describes.

(A) Immunofluorescence
(B) Enzyme immunoassay
(C) Radioimmunoassay
(D) Radial immunodiffusion
(E) Immunoelectrophoresis

C 54. Required to use antibodies labeled with isotopes

A 55. Used to identify antigens in cell walls or membranes

D 56. Used to quantitate immunoglobulin levels in serum

Questions 57–60

Match the characteristic of a definable fragment of degraded immunoglobulin with the most appropriate fragment.

(A) Fab
(B) $F(ab')_2$
(C) Fc
(D) Fd
(E) Fe

A 57. Monovalent fragment that binds antigen

C 58. Fragment that fixes complement

B 59. Formed by pepsin treatment

D 60. V_H and C_H1 domains of heavy (H) chain

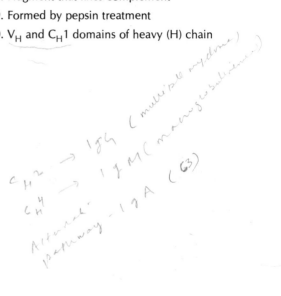

ANSWERS AND EXPLANATIONS

1. The answer is C. (*Chapter 5 IV A 3*) Immunologic memory (anamnesis) is an important characteristic of the immune response. It allows booster shots 5 to 7 years after a primary immunization. More importantly, the rapid rise in antibody levels after re-exposure to a particular infectious agent is responsible for long-lasting convalescent immunity.

2. The answer is B. (*Chapter 9 II D 1–4*) Atopy refers to an immediate hypersensitivity response that occurs only in genetically predisposed hosts upon sensitization to specific allergens. The most direct method of managing atopic allergies is through environmental control (i.e., avoidance of the specific allergen or allergens responsible for the allergic reaction). Other forms of management include immunotherapy, which can be accomplished through hyposensitization or administration of modified allergens, and drug treatment (e.g., with antihistamines, corticosteroids, or epinephrine).

3. The answer is A. (*Chapter 1 II E 1 a, 2 b*) Natural killer (NK) cells are involved in tumor rejection and in reactions to virally infected cells and perhaps some other parasitic states; however, they are not involved in graft rejection. Graft rejection and tumor rejection share the feature of cytotoxic T (Tc)-cell activity and antibody, coupled with either complement, macrophages, or killer (K) cells. The latter cells are also referred to as antibody-dependent cellular cytotoxic (ADCC) cells.

4. The answer is D. (*Chapter 13 III C 1–3*) The principles of immunotherapy of human tumors include the reduction of tumor load by surgery, chemotherapy, or both; modification of tumor cells to enhance antigenicity and eliminate viability; and activation of the immune response via adjuvants. The use of viable tumor cells for specific immunization of the patient should not be attempted, as the possible presence of oncogenic viruses in the vaccine presents a major threat to the recipient.

5. The answer is D. (*Chapter 2 I C 1–5*) The sites on antigens with which antibodies react are called epitopes. These will comprise approximately three to four amino acids, or three to four monosaccharide units. They will be distributed throughout the surface of the antigen and appear in a repeating manner, such that any particular epitope will appear on the antigen surface six or more times. In addition, any particular antigen will likely have different epitopes, such that there may be seven different immunologically specific epitopes on an antigen such as bovine serum albumin. This array of epitopes is referred to as the epitope or determinant group mosaic of an antigen. The total number of epitopes on a particular antigen will be equal to the valence of that antigen, that is, the number of antibody molecules with which that particular antigen could potentially react.

6. The answer is D. [*Chapter 6 II B 2 c (1), (2)*] Antibodies may inhibit an immune response by cytolytic action on the cells of that immune response. Thus, antiserum against antigen-presenting macrophages or B cells or T cells would interfere with immune responses. Antibodies also can interfere with immune responses by interfering with the sensitization phase. For example, RhoGAM suppresses Rh sensitization by diverting the antigen into a catabolic pathway of phagocytosis and destruction rather than a "processing" and "presentation" route to the induction of immunoglobulin synthesis. Antibody can react with an antigen and enhance that antigen's phagocytosis and intracellular destruction, thus preventing its triggering of B cells into proliferation and differentiation into antibody-forming plasma cells. Neutrophils are not antigen-processing cells; hence, they have no role in the immune response.

7. The answer is E. (*Chapter 1 II E 1 d; Chapter 12 VI B 3 d, e*) In order for effective induction of an immune response to occur, the component cells (macrophages, T cells, and B cells) must be identical at the class II major histocompatibility (MHC) locus. The D/DR locus codes for the cell membrane antigens sometimes called Ia (for immune response-associated). Cellular interactions in the effector arm of the immune response have class I MHC restriction. Natural killer (NK) and killer (K) cells do not have any MHC restriction.

8. The answer is E. (*Chapter 4 II A 1 a*) Activation of complement may occur via either the classical or the alternative pathway. The classical pathway may be activated by antigen–antibody complexes involving, primarily, IgG or IgM. In the case of IgG, activation follows binding of complement to the C_H2 domain on the Fc fragment. With IgM, complement binds to the C_H4 domain.

9. The answer is D. (*Chapter 12 II B*) In order to function in graft recognition, histocompatibility antigens must be accessible to the cells of the immune system (i.e., they must be located at the suface of the cell). Class I antigens are glycoproteins in noncovalent association with a β_2-microglobulin. They are found on all nucleated cells of the body. Class II antigens are found on the surfaces of macrophages, T cells, and B cells. They are composed of two membrane-inserted, glycosylated proteins, alpha and beta, which are noncovalently bonded. The major histocompatibility complex antigens in man are called human leukocyte antigens (HLAs) and are coded for by genes on chromosome 6.

10. The answer is B. (*Chapter 2 I A 1, 2 a, b*) Antigenicity is defined as the capacity of a molecule to react with the immunologic product that it induced (i.e., either a humoral antibody or a sensitized lymphocyte). This term is also often used to describe a molecule that can induce an immune response. However, it is probably more accurate to use the term "immunogenic" to describe molecules that are able to induce immune responses. Affinity and avidity are terms which describe the strength of interaction between an antigen and its homologous antibody.

11. The answer is A. (*Chapter 5 V A 1, 2 a–c; Chapter 12 II B 3 a*) Macrophage and neutrophil membranes contain receptors for the Fc fragment of IgG and IgM (but not IgE) as well as for the complement activation product C3b. These receptors are involved in the process of opsonization (i.e., sensitization of foreign material to phagocytosis). In addition, the macrophage contains in its membrane molecules referred to as immune response-associated (Ia) antigens. These are products of genes that occur in the major histocompatibility complex (MHC) of the chromosome and are involved in interaction of the macrophage with lymphoid cells in the immune response; most particularly, the interaction between the macrophage as the antigen-processing cell and the B cell as the precursor of the antibody-producing plasma cell. In the human, they are referred to as class II antigens and are coded for by genes occurring at the D/DR locus.

12. The answer is C. (*Chapter 3 IV A 2*) Idiotypes represent unique amino acid sequences in the variable (V) region of immunoglobulin molecules, which are associated with the antigen-binding capability of the molecule. They are usually specific for the individual antibody clone.

13. The answer is B. (*Chapter 12 I D; III A; IV A 1*) The most important antigenic system in organ transplantation is the ABO system. An organ from a donor who has either the A or B antigens must not be transplanted to a recipient who has anti-A or anti-B isoagglutinins. This incompatibility causes hyperacute or accelerated graft rejection. In some instances, the graft will not even be vascularized. The human leukocyte antigen (HLA) system is also important in evaluation for organ transplantation. Usually, there are not preformed antibodies against HLA antigens except in multiparous women and in persons who may have received numerous transfusions or grafts at a previous time. Sensitization to these antigens is a slower process, and graft rejection may take weeks to months.

14. The answer is A. [*Chapter 6 II B 2 c (2); Chapter 9 III C 1 b*] Erythroblastosis fetalis can be prevented in a future pregnancy by injecting RhoGAM into an Rh-negative mother shortly after delivery of an Rh-positive infant. RhoGAM is an antibody specific to the $RH_0(D)$ antigen—the antigen that induces erythroblastosis. If the mother is Rh-negative and carrying an Rh-positive fetus, some of the fetal red blood cells bearing the RH_0 antigen can cross the placenta and enter the mother's circulation (most frequently during delivery). Once sensitized, the mother will produce antibodies to the antigen, which can cross the placenta during a subsequent pregnancy and damage the fetus. RhoGAM blocks the induction of anti-Rh_0 antibody production in the mother. RhoGAM cannot be given prior to delivery as it would cross the placenta and cause damage to the fetus.

15. The answer is B. (*Chapter 7 IV B, C 1–4*) Hepatitis A (infectious hepatitis or short incubation hepatitis) immune globulin is an example of a human-derived immune globulin (IG) that is prepared from normal adult human plasma or serum and is used for passive immunization against certain diseases or for maintenance of immunodeficient persons; it is not a specific immune globulin (SIG). SIG is a gamma globulin obtained from hyperimmunized human volunteers or from individuals who have recently recovered from a specific infectious disease such as rabies, varicella (chickenpox), or tetanus. Rh immune globulin is a hyperimmune preparation used in Rh-negative women within 72 hours of delivery, miscarriage, or abortion of an Rh-positive baby or fetus to prevent sensitization of the mother to possible Rh-positive red blood cells in future pregnancies.

16. The answer is B. [*Chapter 8 IV B 2 b (1) (a); Chapter 11 I*] The presence of a positive mumps skin test suggests that the patient has intact T-cell immunity. The ability of the serum to cause hemolysis of antibody-sensitized erythrocytes indicates that the complement system is functioning. Phagocytic function tests of chemotaxis and intracellular killing suggest that the phagocytes are also functioning normally in this patient. A positive Schick test indicates that the individual is unable to mount a humoral immune response, which is a B-cell immunodeficiency. If the patient had produced antibodies to the diphtheria toxin, the toxin would have been neutralized and no inflammatory reaction would have occurred at the site of injection.

17. The answer is E. [*Chapter 3 II C, D, E 1 a, b; Chapter 8 II C 2 a–c (1)–(3)*] It may help to resolve this dilemma by referring to the chapter on antibody structure. Antibody to gamma chains will have antibodies specific to V_H, C_H1, C_H2, and C_H3 domains; hence, all the reactions discussed (and illustrated) will occur. If, however, the center well contained antibodies to light chains, there would be no reaction with Fd (line 3–4) nor Fc (line 4–1). The spur at 2 would also disappear.

18. The answer is C. (*Chapter 6 II B 1 c*) Cancer chemotherapy involves the inhibition of cell division. As immune responses depend upon proliferation of lymphoid cells, drugs that block DNA replication or cause errors in the process will be immunosuppressive. This action will predispose the individual to infections, commonly by agents not normally considered to be pathogenic (opportunists). This is true because these organisms are often normal flora or common environmental contacts and will take advantage of the depressed state of the host to invade, multiply, and produce disease.

19. The answer is E. (*Chapter 11 V C*) Wiskott-Aldrich syndrome consists of a triad of features including thrombocytopenia, which is usually present at birth; eczema, which is usually present at the age of 1 year; and recurrent pyogenic infection starting after the age of 6 months. Immunologic abnormalities suggest combined B- and T-cell defects. The defect in antibody response to polysaccharide antigens renders the patients susceptible to infection with capsular polysaccharide-type organisms (e.g., *Streptococcus pneumoniae*, *Neisseria meningitidis*, and *Haemophilus influenzae*). Death is usually due to bleeding problems (thrombocytopenia) or sepsis or both.

20. The answer is D. (*Chapter 7 IV B*) Immune globulin (IG), also called gamma globulin, is prepared from pooled normal adult human plasma or serum by cold ethanol fractionation. The primary antibody to diseases in IG is IgG. IG is one of three basic types of serum preparations used to induce passive artificially acquired immunity, the other two being antitoxin and specific immune globulin (SIG).

21. The answer is E. [*Chapter 9 III C 1 a (1), (2)*] Transfusion reactions can be classified as immunologic or nonimmunologic. Immunologically mediated transfusion reactions are important clinical examples of cytotoxic (type II) reactions and can occur by two different mechanisms—rapid intravascular hemolysis of red blood cells or extravascular destruction of antibody-sensitized red blood cells, primarily by the cells of the reticuloendothelial system (RES). Transfusion reactions that are due to intravascular hemolysis are characterized by anti-A or anti-B antibodies binding to complement, with almost immediate lysis of transfused red blood cells. Transfusion reactions that are due to extravascular hemolysis almost invariably are involved with Rh incompatibility and are not complement mediated. IgE is crucial to the pathogenesis of immediate hypersensitivity (type I) reactions; IgE is not involved in cytotoxic reactions.

22. The answer is A. (*Chapter 6 III B 6 a–c*) Immune tolerance is most easily induced in T cells and will have a longer duration in these lymphocytes than it will in B cells. It takes less antigen to induce tolerance in T cells, and the tolerance occurs within 1 day of exposure to antigen in contrast to B cells, where tolerance will take 4 to 5 days to become established. Macrophages do not have antigenic specificity and hence are not rendered immunologically tolerant.

23. The answer is C. (*Chapter 9 III A, B*) The same immunologic mechanisms that defend the host at times may cause severe damage to tissues. These damaging immunologic reactions (also called hypersensitivity reactions) have been classified into four types according to the mechanism of tissue injury. Immediate hypersensitivity (type I) reactions are initiated by antigen reacting with cell-bound antibody—usually IgE. Cytotoxic (type II) reactions are initiated by antibody—usually IgG or IgM—reacting with cell-bound antigen. Immune complex–mediated (type III) reactions are initiated by antigen–antibody complexes that form locally or are deposited from the circulation. Delayed hypersensitivity (cell-mediated; type IV) reactions are initiated by sensitized (antigen-reactive) T cells reacting with specific antigens. A fifth mechanism of tissue injury has been identified (sometimes referred to as a ''type V reaction''), in which antibody interferes with the functioning of biologically active substances (e.g., clotting factors and intrinsic factors).

24. The answer is B. (*Chapter 8 II E 1, 2*) Syphilis serology, using serum specimens collected serially from pregnant women and from infants following delivery, is of value in diagnosing congenital syphilis. The syphilitic host develops, among other antibodies, an antibody (reagin) to a nontreponemal antigen (beef heart cardiolipin). Reagin may be found in both serum and spinal fluid and it forms readily visible clumps when it combines with cardiolipin in what is referred to as a flocculation test. The Venereal Disease Research Laboratory (VDRL) and rapid plasma reagin (RPR) tests are practical and simple to perform. Although these tests are not specific for syphilis, they are extremely sensitive and useful.

25. The answer is E. (*Chapter 3 III C 2 a*) A pregnant syphilitic woman can transmit the causative microorganism, *Treponema pallidum*, to her fetus through the placenta beginning at about the 10th to 16th week of gestation. If therapy is not instituted the fetus may die in utero, the infected newborn may die shortly after delivery, or, as in the case presented in the question, the infant may survive but develop signs of congenital syphilis later. Rapid diagnosis of congenitally acquired syphilis in live newborns is essential, but it may be difficult if based only on clinical findings since many infected infants may be asymptomatic at birth. Certain intrauterine infections of the fetus lead to elevated IgM levels as demonstrated in cord serum at birth or in the postnatal period. Since maternal IgM does not normally cross the placenta, the IgM level in the newborn is a reflection of antigenic stimulation during the intra-uterine period. The normal IgM level in cord serum is approximately 10 mg/dl. Concentrations above about 20 mg/dl may be seen in syphilitic newborns who are totally asymptomatic at birth and remain so for variable periods. Screening of cord and newborn serum for IgM elevation can be of more diagnostic value in these types of infections than determination of Venereal Disease Research Laboratory (VDRL) titer. It should be emphasized, however, that an increase in IgM is not, per se, enough to establish the exact nature of the infection (i.e., the identity of the etiologic agent).

26. The answer is E (all). [*Chapter 11 II B 1 a (1), (2)*] Chronic granulomatous disease is an immunodeficiency syndrome with onset in the first 2 years of life; it is inherited primarily as an X-linked trait. Characteristics include recurrent bacterial infections, hepatosplenomegaly, lymphadenopathy, and granuloma formation, which appears to reflect faulty phagocytosis. Neutrophils fail to respond to phagocytosis with the normal oxidative burst apparently due to a reduction in the level of intracellular reduced nicotinamide adenine dinucleotide (NADH) or nicotinamide adenine dinucleotide phosphate (NADPH).

27. The answer is C (2, 4). (*Chapter 1 II D 1 a, 2 b, c, E 3*) Beta lysin and properdin are proteins that contribute to natural immunity. Beta lysin is an antibacterial protein released from blood platelets when they rupture, as in clot formation, and it is active primarily against gram-positive bacteria. Properdin is a protein different from normal antibody and complement but believed to work in conjunction with the two (plus magnesium ions) to effect bactericidal action. Properdin is involved in complement activation by the alternative pathway. Bacteriolysis occurs due to the lytic action of antibody-activated complement on the outer lipopolysaccharide layer of the cell wall, while lymphokine activated killer (LAK) cells are naturally occurring cytotoxic lymphocytes.

28. The answer is E (all). (*Chapter 12 II B 1, 3 e*) Genes that influence response to many antigens [immune response (Ir) genes] are associated with the HLA locus D/DR. Antibody formation is not stimulated by Ir genes through direct action on B cells, rather the genes appear to act by effecting cellular interaction between B cells and T cells, and antigen-presenting cells such as macrophages.

29. The answer is C (2, 4). (*Chapter 9 II B 3 b, d–f*) Immediate hypersensitivity (type I) reactions involve the release of pharmacologically active substances (mediators) from mast cells or basophils, a mechanism that is triggered by antigens reacting with preformed, cell-bound IgE. The mediators of type I are classified as either preformed or formed upon initiation of the immediate hypersensitivity response. Mediators that exist preformed in mediator cells include histamine (probably the most important of these substances), eosinophil chemotactic factor of anaphylaxis (ECF-A), and serotonin (5-hydroxytryptamine). Mediators that form and are released after the antigen–antibody reaction include slow-reacting substance of anaphylaxis (SRS-A), platelet-activating factor (PAF), bradykinin, and prostaglandins.

30. The answer is D (4). (*Chapter 9 V B 3*) Delayed hypersensitivity is induced by uptake of antigen by macrophages and activation of T cells. Induction requires that the cells not only recognize immunogenic epitopes but also class II determinants of the major histocompatibility complex (MHC) gene products. Interaction between antigen-processing cells and T cells can only occur if the two participants are MHC identical. Under the influence of antigen and MHC gene products, the T cells become antigen-reactive (activated, sensitized).

31. The answer is E (all). (*Chapter 3 III C*) IgM has a pentameric structure consisting of five basic units linked by J chain and disulfide bonds at the Fc fragment. The basic units contain $\varkappa$ or λ light chains and μ heavy chains. A preparation of pooled human IgM would be expected to be antigenic for the rabbit and to induce the formation of antibodies reactive with the individual immunoglobulin components.

32. The answer is E (all). (*Chapter 10 V D, F, G, H*) Systemic lupus erythematosus (SLE) is a possible diagnosis for the patient presented in the question. On occasion, this disease can affect the central nervous system (CNS). However, the fact that the patient had been well up to the time of the present illness tends to rule out SLE as does the predilection of the disease for young women. Myasthenia gravis and multiple sclerosis are possible diagnoses, although the rapid onset of a near-fatal disease tends to exclude these. The patient in this case has Guillain-Barré syndrome.

33. The answer is E (all). (*Chapter 10 V D 2 b, F 2, G 2 a, H b*) Indirect immunofluorescence can detect antinuclear antibodies in the sera of patients with systemic lupus erythematosus (SLE). A positive test for antinuclear antibodies is necessary for the diagnosis of SLE in a young or middle-aged woman. Obviously, an immunofluorescence test for antinuclear antibodies can be positive in the presence of other diseases, such as rheumatoid arthritis and scleroderma, and in cases in which there is a history of drug ingestion; these factors must be first ruled out. The diagnosis of multiple sclerosis is contingent upon the clinical features of the disease. However, most patients with multiple sclerosis will have abnormalities on laboratory tests. One of the most dependable indications is a finding of an increase in IgG in the spinal fluid of patients. IgG values often are normal early in the course of multiple sclerosis. The increase in IgG levels is highest in cases of the greatest duration and in the face of severe neurologic deficits. The most important autoimmune feature of myasthenia gravis is the presence of antibodies to the human acetylcholine receptor. The majority (approximately 80%–85%) of patients with myasthenia gravis have abnormally high serum levels of these antibodies. Antinervous tissue antibodies can be detected in Guillain-Barre patient serum by complement fixation test procedures.

34. The answer is D (4). *(Chapter 10 V F)* A lumbar puncture was performed to rule out encephalomyelitis. This procedure should not be done in the case of a brain abscess as the intracranial pressure may be great enough to cause downward displacement of the brain. An elevated white blood count would suggest an infectious process. Neutrophils predominate if the cause is bacterial; lymphocytes predominate if the cause is viral. Glucose levels are also usually depleted if the disease is of bacterial origin. An elevated protein content coupled with otherwise normal cerebrospinal fluid findings is suggestive of Guillain-Barré syndrome.

35. The answer is A (1, 2, 3). *(Chapter 2 I B 2; II A)* The recommendations of the staff immunologist to the director of the radioimmunoassay laboratory should include increasing the number of animals to at least three. Rabbits are random-bred animals and will not respond uniformly to an immunization procedure. By increasing the number of animals, the chances of finding one high responder increases. The route of administration and the dosage of the antibiotic are fine. Gentamicin is a hapten, and it is not likely to induce any immune response. The probability of its coupling to carrier proteins in the rabbit is extremely small. This problem could be bypassed by chemically conjugating the antibiotic to a carrier molecule before injection. Foreignness is important in immunogenicity; therefore, bovine serum albumin is recommended. An even better vehicle might be human erythrocytes. They are not only foreign to the rabbit but have additional attributes of greater chemical complexity and phagocytizability. (If phagocyte interaction is deemed important, the intravenous route of injection would probably be more suitable.)

36. The answer is C (2, 4). *(Chapter 8 V B)* The many assays that are available for detecting immune complexes in serum can be divided into three types: solid phase binding assays, fluid phase binding assays, and cellular binding assays. The reaction of immune complexes with complement allows for many ways to detect immune complexes. For example, complement-fixing immune complexes can be detected by direct measurement of the binding of immune complexes to C1q; this can be done using a solid phase or a fluid phase binding assay. The interaction of complement-coated immune complexes with complement receptors on cells (e.g., Raji cells) also may be used; the Raji cell binding assay is an example of a cellular binding assay. The radioallergosorbent (RAST) test is used to assay specific IgE levels in vitro, the Prausnitz-Küstner (PK) reaction is an in vivo passive transfer test used to assay specific IgE in serum.

37. The answer is D (4). *[Chapter 13 II B 1 b (1), (2), (3)]* Carcinoembryonic antigen (CEA) is associated with carcinoma of the colon and pancreas; however, because CEA also occurs in nonmalignant conditions (e.g., cigarette smoking), it is not considered to be diagnostic of but merely suggestive of a cancerous condition. Assays for CEA show their greatest promise in follow-up for the recurrence of certain malignancies.

38. The answer is B (1, 3). *[Chapter 13 II B 1 b (1)]* The presence of carcinoembryonic antigen (CEA) in the serum is correlated with the severity of certain malignant and nonmalignant states or with the tumor burden of the host. The higher the level of CEA, the greater the tumor mass is in the patient. Following surgical excision of the tumor, the CEA level should drop to very low or perhaps indiscernible levels. If the CEA level rises again, it suggests that the tumor has metastasized and appropriate therapeutic or surgical intervention is indicated. The patient presented is gravely ill. Surgical removal of the tumor was incomplete and metastases have developed as indicated by the rise in CEA in months 10–12. The chemotherapeutic regimen should be reevaluated and the patient should be thoroughly examined for possible radiologic and surgical treatment.

39. The answer is A (1, 2, 3). *(Chapter 8 II A, C, D 2; III A)* Tests that could be used to detect tetanus antitoxin include toxin neutralization, complement fixation, and precipitation. Toxin neutralization would require the use of animals or tissue cultures and, hence, may be beyond the means of most laboratories. Complement fixation is an acceptable alternate; however, it requires the pretitration of the component reagents, which would necessitate the purchase of a standardized tetanus antitoxin. The simplest, although not the most sensitive, assay would be precipitation, either in solution or in an agar medium. The advantage of the latter is economy of reagents, as several serum samples could be assayed against the same toxoid preparation in an Ouchterlony plate technique. Agglutination would not be of any value because the toxin is excreted and is not cell-bound. Passive hemagglutination in which the antigen (tetanus toxoid) is adsorbed to a red blood cell carrier would be an excellent assay.

40. The answer is E (all). (*Chapter 8 II A 3 a, b; III A, B 2; IV A 2*) Antibodies to the typhoid bacillus are conveniently titrated by tube or slide agglutination procedures. A classic example of the application of the agglutination reaction is seen in the Widal test in the diagnosis of typhoid fever. Bactericidal assay, complement fixation, and indirect immunofluorescence techniques could also be employed; however, all of these procedures are considerably more complex and time-consuming and would not be the test of choice.

41. The answer is A (1, 2, 3). (*Chapter 11 III D 2; IV A 2; V B 1, C 1*) Normal recovery from viral diseases suggests an intact thymus-dependent immune system, thus eliminating DiGeorge, Nezelof's, and Wiskott-Aldrich syndromes, all of which feature variable or total deficits in T-cell immunity. Selective immunoglobulin deficiency could be considered due to its characteristic of normal T-cell function.

42. The answer is E (all). (*Chapter 11 II A 1 c, B 1, 4, 5*) The normal leukocyte differential count would exclude the de Vaal syndrome, which is characterized by a diminished production of phagocytic cells. Normal leukocytic function would not be characteristic of chronic granulomatous disease (impaired intracellular killing), Job's syndrome (faulty chemotactic responses), or the lazy leukocyte syndrome (defective chemotactic response and abnormal inflammatory response).

43. The answer is D (4). (*Chapter 11 III A 1, C 1, D 2; V C 1, 3*) The patient has Bruton's hypogammaglobulinemia. The presence of a small amount of IgG is consistent with this diagnosis. Common variable hypogammaglobulinemia resembles Bruton's disease, except that symptoms first appear in patients aged 20–30 years. Selective immunoglobulin deficiency is characterized by a decrease in serum level of one or more immunoglobulin classes, with selective IgA deficiency being the most common form (i.e., little serum IgA but normal or increased levels of IgG and IgM). Wiskott-Aldrich syndrome features low IgM, elevated IgA and IgE, but normal IgG levels.

44–47. The answers are: 44-A, 45-A, 46-B, 47-C. (*Chapter 1 II C 5 a; Chapter 3 I, III C, D; Chapter 12 II B 2 b, 3 a*) B cells can be quantitated in peripheral blood by determining the number of cells which form EAC rosettes. EAC cells are erythrocytes that have antibody and complement on their membrane. B cells contain a receptor for C3b which will react with that complement activation product on the erythrocyte and will cause those erythrocytes to adhere to the B-cell membrane. They will then form a mulberry-shaped aggregate called a rosette. These can be counted microscopically.

T cells are primarily involved in graft rejection. Human leukocyte antigen (HLA)-A and HLA-B are the principal antigen products of the major histocompatibility complex (MHC) recognized by the host during the process of graft rejection. In cell-mediated cytolysis (CMC), the in vitro correlate of graft rejection, HLA-A and HLA-B antigens are the target antigens recognized by the cytotoxic T (Tc) cells.

Class II MHC antigen restriction occurs among the macrophage, B cell, and T cell, indicating that the macrophage, B cell, and T cell must have the same class II histocompatibility antigen on their membranes to interact. Class I MHC antigens are involved in effector cell recognition events. IgM and IgD are the first antibodies made in utero. They first can be seen in the cytoplasm of B cells. Later in development, they will appear as a part of the membrane. They are the external expression of the immunologic commitment (specificity) of the cell.

48. The answer is C. [*Chapter 12 II C 1 b (1); IV A 1*] Acute or accelerated graft rejection is due to sensitized lymphocytes. Multiparity would induce both humoral and cellular sensitization. Blood group incompatibility is strictly an antibody-mediated event, and it is the cause of hyperacute rejection.

49. The answer is D. [*Chapter 8 IV B 2 b (2)*] Individuals of blood group AB do not have isohemagglutinins in their plasma; if they did they would have some type of hemolytic disease. Individuals of blood group O will have both anti-A and anti-B isohemagglutinins in their plasma. An individual of blood group A will have anti-B, and blood group B individuals will have anti-A isohemagglutinins.

50–53. The answers are: 50-D, 51-E, 52-B, 53-E. [*Chapter 3 III A 2 c, B 1 b (1), C 2 b; Chapter 4 II A 1 a*] The complement system, which plays a major role in host defense and the inflammatory process, can be activated via the classical and alternative pathways. Activation of the pathways may occur via antigen–antibody complexes or by aggregated immunoglobulins. IgG molecules (mainly the IgG_1, IgG_2, and IgG_3 subclasses) are capable of fixing complement. Activation of the classical pathway follows binding of complement to the C_H2 domain site on the Fc fragment of IgG. Serum IgA fixes complement via the alternative pathway only. Activation of this pathway can be triggered immunologically primarily by IgA (and to a lesser degree by some IgG). IgM is the most efficient immunoglobulin at fixing complement via the classical pathway. Only one molecule of IgM is required to react with complement. Activation of the classical pathway follows binding of complement to the C_H4 domain site on the Fc fragment of IgM.

54–56. The answers are: 54-C, 55-A, 56-D. (*Chapter 8 II C 3; III B 1, G*) Radioimmunoassay procedures are extremely sensitive measures of either antigen or antibody. The amplification step, which gives these such great sensitivity, is the utilization of radioactive isotopes coupled to the compound being detected. Thus, a very small amount of antigen or antibody can be detected because of its high radioactivity. Commonly iodine 125(^{125}I) is employed as the radioactive isotope label.

In the immunofluorescence technique, antibody to a particular bacterium, cell membrane, or cytoplasm constituent is labeled with a fluorescent dye, usually fluorescein. Once the antibody has reacted with the organism or tissue component, the excess gamma globulin is removed by washing the slide, which is examined in an ultraviolet light microscope. Fluorescein emits energy when excited by ultraviolet wavelength rays and emits light in the green wavelengths so that, where that fluorescein molecule is (i.e., where the antibody is), an apple-green appearance will be seen in the dark-field microscope.

Radial immunodiffusion is employed to quantitate immunoglobulin levels in serum as well as levels of other serum proteins such as the complement components, alpha-1-trypsin inhibitor, and others. In this test, the antigen in question diffuses out into an agar menstruum which is impregnated with specific antibodies. A precipitant ring will develop. The diameter of that ring is directly proportional to the amount of antigen placed in the well. Thus, by the appropriate utilization of known samples, it is possible to quantitate the amount of a serum protein in an unknown specimen.

57–60. The answers are: 57-A, 58-C, 59-B, 60-D. (*Chapter 3 II E 1 a, b, 2*) Treatment of the monomeric basic immunoglobulin unit with papain splits it into two monovalent Fab (antigen-binding) fragments and one Fc (crystallizable) fragment.

Pepsin treatment of the immunoglobulin molecule digests away most of the Fc fragment, leaving two Fab fragments and the hinge region, termed an F(ab')$_2$ fragment, which is bivalent.

The Fc fragment that is produced by papain digestion of immunoglobulin contains the carboxy terminal half of the heavy (H) chain. It is the site for complement binding.

Each Fab fragment derived from papain digestion of immunoglobulin contains an entire light chain plus the V$_H$ and C$_H$1 domains of the heavy chain (the Fd fragment).

Index

Note: Page numbers in *italics* denote illustrations; those followed by (t) denote tables; those followed by Q denote questions; and those followed by E denote explanations.

Bacterial cell virulence factor, 26
Bacterial meningitis vaccine, 74, 77
Bacterial vaccines, 73–74
Bacteriolysis, 17, 84
Bagassosis, 103
Basic protein of myelin, 25
Basophil, 105
BCG, *see* Bacille Calmette-Guérin
Bence-Jones protein, 105
Benign monoclonal gammopathy, 106
Beta lysin, 17, 156Q, 164E
Bis-diazotized benzidine, 88
Blastogenesis assay, 134–135
Blocking factors, 146
Blood group antigens, inheritance and expression
    of, 135, 135(t)
Body temperature, immunologic function of, 14
Bone-marrow–derived lymphocytes, *see* B cell(s)
Bone marrow transplant, in severe combined
    immunodeficiency disease, 2Q, 8E
Booster immunization, 91
Booster immune response, 52
Bordetella pertussis, as adjuvant, 66, 67(t)
Botulism antitoxin, 75
Bradykinin, 100
Bruton's hypogammaglobulinemia, 1Q, 7E, 63,
    124, 159Q, 166E
Bullous diseases, 102, 117–118
Bullous pemphigoid, 102, 117–118
Bursa-derived lymphocytes, *see* B cell(s)
Bursa of Fabricius, 3Q, 9E, 50, 61

C

C1, in complement activation, 42–43, 42(t)
C1 esterase, 1Q, 7E, 43
C1 esterase inhibitor, deficiency of, 127
C1q, deficiency of, 127
C1q liquid-phase binding assay, 93, 157Q, 165E
C1q solid-phase binding assay, 4Q, 9E, 93, 157Q,
    165E
C2, biological functions of, 46
 in complement activation, 42(t), 43
 deficiency of, 127
C3, biological functions of, 45–46
 in complement activation, 42(t), 43–44
  by classical pathway, 42(t), 43
 deficiency of, 128
C3 convertase, 43, 44
 amplification, 44
C3 nephritic factor, 46
C3 proactivator, 43
C3 proactivator convertase, 43
C3b, 17
C3b inactivator, 43
C4, biological functions of, 46
 in complement activation, 42(t), 43
 deficiency of, 127
C4 binding protein, 45
C4b2a3b complex, 43, 44
C5, biological functions of, 45–46
 in complement activation, 42(t), 44
 deficiency of, 128
C5 convertase, 43, 44
C5a, 17
C5b67 complex, 17, 46
C6, in complement activation, 42(t), 44
 deficiency of, 128
C7, in complement activation, 42(t), 44
C8, in complement activation, 42(t), 45

deficiency of, 128
C9, in complement activation, 42(t), 45
Cachectin, 146
Calcium ions, in complement activation, 42
Cancer, *see also* Tumor(s)
 chemotherapy for, goals of, 153Q, 161E
  immunosuppressive effects of, 62–63, 155Q,
   163E
 immunosuppression in, 63
 post-transplantation, 137
Candidiasis, chronic mucocutaneous, 125–126
Capsular antigens, 26
Carcinoembryonic antigen (CEA), 5Q, 11E, 144,
    158Q, 165E
Cardiolipin, 24, 25
 in VDRL test, 86–87
Carrier molecules, for haptens, 23
Catalase, 16
CD antigens, 54
Cell lysis, *see* Cytolysis
Cell-mediated immunity, 3Q, 9E, 13
 see also Immunity
 and delayed hypersensitivity, 104–105
Chédiak-Higashi syndrome, 124
Chemiluminescence, 17
Chemotaxins, 15
Chemotaxis, 14–15
 assay, 90
 measurement of, 16
Chemotherapy, cancer, goals of, 153Q, 161E
 immunosuppressive effects of, 62–63
Chronic granulomatous disease, 123–124, 156Q,
    159Q, 164E, 166E
 phagocytic dysfunction in, 16
 tests for, 90
Cilia, function of, 14
Classical pathway, *see* Complement
    system, activation of, components of
Clonal deletion theory, 64
Clone, forbidden, 64
Cobra venom factor, 44
Coccidioidomycosis, immunosuppression in, 127
Codominant gene, 132, *132*
Cold antibody hemolytic anemia, 116–117
Collaboration, B-cell and T-cell, 50
Common pathway, *see* Complement system,
    activation of, components of
Common variable hypogammaglobulinemia, 125
Compartmentalization, in immune response system,
    50
Complement fixation test, 84, 87, 160Q, 166E
Complement split products, 17
Complement system, 41–46
 activation of, pathways of, 41–45
  alternative (properdin), 43–44, *44*
  classical, 41–43, *43*
  membrane attack (common), 44–45
  regulation of, 45
 components of, *see also specific components*
  alternative pathway, 43–44
  classical pathway, 42–43
  deficiency of, 127–128
  membrane attack pathway, 44–45
  nomenclature for, 41
  properties of, 42(t)
  and tumor cell lysis, 146
 cytotoxic function of, 41
 inactivators of, 45
 inflammatory function of, 41
 inhibitors of, 45
 opsonic function of, 17, 41
Complete Freund's adjuvant, 66, 67(t)